CURIOSITIES OF THE CONTACT LENS

CURIOSITIES OF THE CONTACT LENS

written by
Richard M. Hill, O.D., Ph.D.
The Ohio State University, Columbus

The Professional Press, Inc.
Chicago, Illinois

FIRST PRINTING
ISBN-0-87873-026-5

Library of Congress Catalog Card Number: 81-80236

Published by The Professional Press, Inc.
Chicago, Illinois 60611

Printed in the U.S.A.

Table of Contents

Part III: THE LENS

The lens as a foreign body: Old and new properties; continuing vulnerabilities; and some of the subtle aspects of care and neglect.

Preface

While already the most cosmetically subtle (and in many ways the most optically effective), the contact lens still retains about it a certain aura of unpredictability—just enough in fact to keep it among the most fascinating challenges of modern ophthalmic practice.

Its lure stems largely from the fundamental challenge to match wits, skill and experience against one of the most formidable arrays of geometric combinations, sets of visual requirements and assorted life styles to be encountered anywhere in the health sciences.

These essays are dedicated specifically to those students and practitioners who not only relish that challenge, but even more so, that special pleasure of tilting the odds just a little more in their favor.

Toward that end, and unlike a comprehensive textbook on the subject, these reviews deal solely with "targets of opportunity," that is clinical problems and curiousities now approachable through continually improving strategies and advancing technology.

As their original references reveal, these explorations, like most science, did not take place in any neat or serial order, but rather as particular ideas or information came to hand. Over some 20 years (including 3 at the University of California, Berkeley), they held the shared interest at one time or anther of a long continuum of students and colleagues, whose enthusiasm and creative efforts have constituted what we've come to call the *Eye Physiology Laboratory* at The Ohio State University College of Optometry.

Special appreciation is expressed here to Dean F.W. Hebbard who fostered an environment so vital to such pursuits, and to Miss Wendy Clark, whose graphics skills added immeasurably to the final result.

RMH

CURIOSITIES OF THE CONTACT LENS

Part 1: THE TEARS

Exploring the lens environment: Tear and solution pH, wettability, salt balance, oxygen content, oily quality and volumes contained under a contact lens.

Chapter One

The pH Mystique

Of the many characteristics of a contact lens system, tear pH has possibly remained the most clinically "intangible." When asked, practitioners will often say that pH seems to have something to do with eye comfort—at least some patients seem to show less tolerance than do others to the pH of certain solutions.

Some practitioners have even attempted a "solution match" of their patient's tears by measuring them with pH indicator strips* and then recommending a solution whose pH is the same. But a "solution match" assumes, of course, that the tears involved have a nearly constant pH value. Can this be true? That is, is a patient's tear pH virtually "immutable"?

Playing the Odds

To search out that answer, over 2000 tear samples have been studied.[1-6] Each sample was collected by gently placing a tiny tube down into the lower conjunctival sac, allowing it to fill passively by capillary action. The tube is then immediately sealed to prevent air contact with the tear

*The use of indicator strips is not recommended for this purpose, however, since the commonly used forms: (1) are not sterile, (2) are possibly toxic due to certain dyes used, and (3) generally give an erroneous answer due to carbon dioxide exchange between the wet strip and the air (producing an answer which is significantly more acid than is correct).

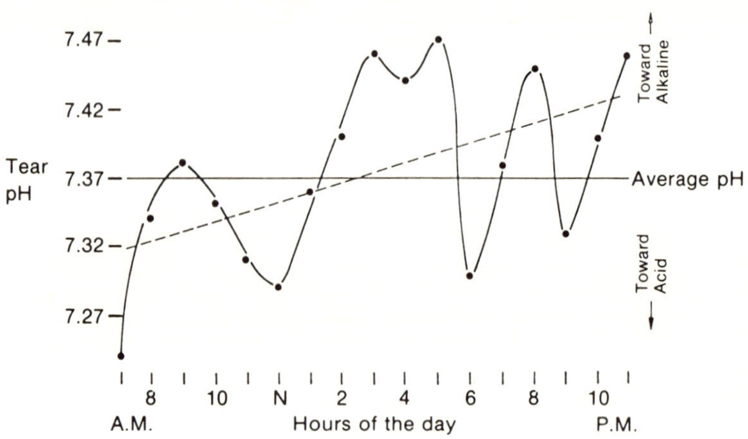

FIGURE 1. Variations in the pH of one patient's tears throughout a day. The broken line represents the rate of progression from the most acid level found on awakening toward more alkaline levels in the course of the day.[3]

sample until it is drawn into a closed, temperature-regulated microelectrode chamber for analysis.

If hourly samples are collected, it is possible to reconstruct a patient's tear pH history throughout the day, as shown for example in Figure 1. But how can we analyze such a complex profile?

This could certainly be done by counting or measuring the several distinctive features of this history, for example, (1) the number of alkaline high points (there are three major ones) and acidic low points (one at awakening, plus three more); (2) the average pH for the waking day (7.37); (3) the frequency of crossing that mean value in the course of the day (seven times); (4) the magnitude of pH swing during the waking day (7.46 to 7.24); or (5) the net shift toward alkalinity as the day progresses (an average rate of 0.008 pH units per hour).

A probability approach might be much more interesting clinically. For example, we could ask what the odds would be (chances out of 100), that a particular patient's tears would be more than 0.1 of a pH unit (a very small drift indeed!) from his average daily value. The shaded zones in Figure 2 show that such a variance happened less than one percent of the time during that patient's day, and that this particular time was in the early morning (observed on just awakening.)[2]

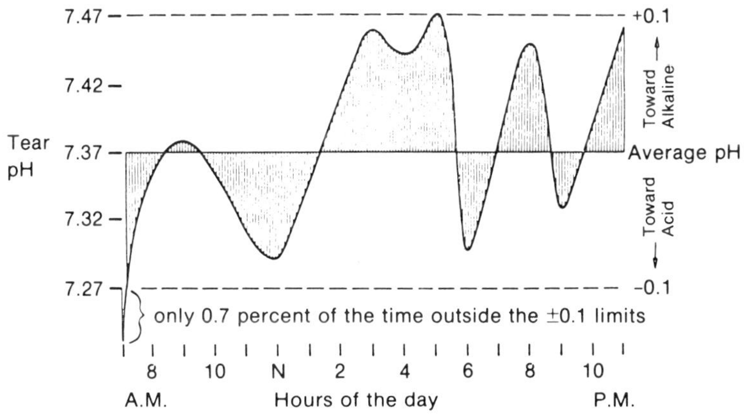

FIGURE 2. A probability approach to describe the variation of tear pH for the same patient described in Figure 1. The shaded time zones represent the 99+ percent part of the day that this patient's tear pH remained within 0.1 of his average value.[3]

Each patient, however, has unique patterns that are not always repeatable even from day to day. One possible explanation for this variation is that tear pH, as well as being subject to the instabilities of the atmospheric environment, may be a reflection as well of similar pH shifts (although of a more limited amplitude) known to take place in the blood.

Impact of a Contact Lens

Although only 13 patients have been studied in detail so far, [4,5] it appears that the daytime wear of contact lenses has only a minor effect (if any) on pH. This fact is especially important in relation to an earlier concern that hydrophilic lenses might accumulate acid byproducts in the course of wear.

The observations described[4,5] give no indication that the tears, at least, are being adversely affected by the presence of these prescription forms.

Overview

Tear pH, then, is a continually changing function of the human eye, but one whose deviations (assuming no pathology) remain within fairly limited bounds, presumably through the presence of natural buffer systems (i.e., proteins, the bicarbonate system). Similarly, the presence of a contact lens, either hard or soft, under waking conditions does not seem to alter significantly tear pH in the healthy eye. Sleep conditions do depress the tear pH somewhat in the average patient (down to about 7.25 vs. 7.45 for the waking hours), but pilot studies[6] with a hydrophilic lens (HEMA) in place overnight did not reveal any further exaggeration of that shift. Larger samples, however, will need to be tested before final conclusions can be reached in that province.

References

1. Carney, L.G. and R.M. Hill, Human tear pH. *Arch. Ophthal.*, 94:821, 1976.
2. Carney, L.G. and R.M. Hill, pH profiles: I. *J. Amer. Optom. Assoc.*, 46:1143, 1975.
3. Hill, R.M. and L. G. Carney, pH profiles: II. *J. Amer. Optom. Assoc.*, 46:1146, 1975.
4. Carney, L.G. and R.M. Hill, Tear pH and the hard (PMMA) contact lens patient. *Intern. Contact Lens Clinic,* 3(2):27, 1976.
5. Hill, R.M. and L.G. Carney, Tear pH and the soft contact lens patient. *Intern. Contact Lens Clinic,* 4(3):71-77, 1977.
6. Carney, L.G. and R.M. Hill, Tear pH: Hydrophilic lenses and the closed eye. *Intern. Contact Lens Clinic,* 3(2):30, 1976.
7. Hastings, A.B. and C.W. Eisele, Diurnal variations in acid-base balance. *Proc. Soc. Exp. Biol. Med.*, 43:308, 1940.

Chapter Two

The World of pH 7

There are several traditional "benchmarks" for gauging eye response. Of these, tear pH probably is the least tangible or predictable. Every patient has highly individual sensitivity thresholds, ranges of daily variation, reactions to lens presence, tolerances to solution acidities, etc.[1-4]

There is little argument that tears should be around pH 7 in order to meet the complex needs of the cornea and to minimize clinical problems. (A recent human tear pH average was 7.45, based on 1,068 open eye samples from 16 young adults[5].) How resistant is tear pH to a spontaneous challenge?

The Ten-To-One Impact

As with anything so familiar, it is easy to forget what a shift of pH actually means. The units used are so powerful that we are ophthalmically obliged to scale them in 10ths and, where experimental controls and reliability permit, even in 100ths.

To appreciate the impact of a change of 1 pH unit, we might use the relative model in Figure 1. A microcosm of neutral (pH 7) tears contains only seven hydrogen ions (i.e., the common acidity-determining particle). Suppose, however, that something were to force our microcosm's pH just 1 unit in the acid direction to a value of 6. As illustrated in the center of Figure 1, such change would be 10-fold increase in the number of

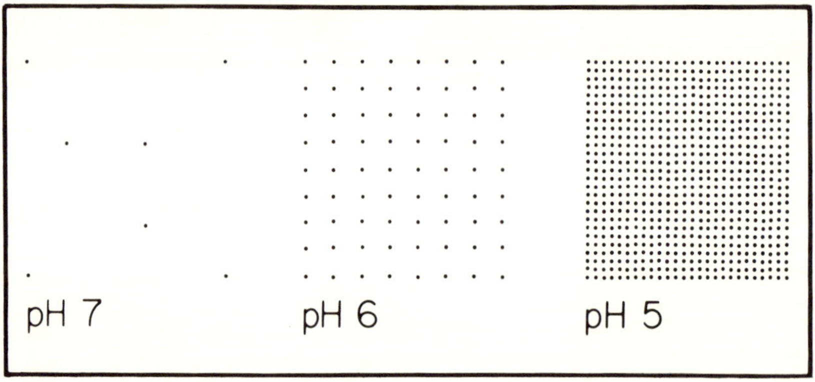

FIGURE 1. Microcosms of ophthalmic solutions containing proportions of hydrogen ions representing a progressively more acid pH of 7, 6 and 5.

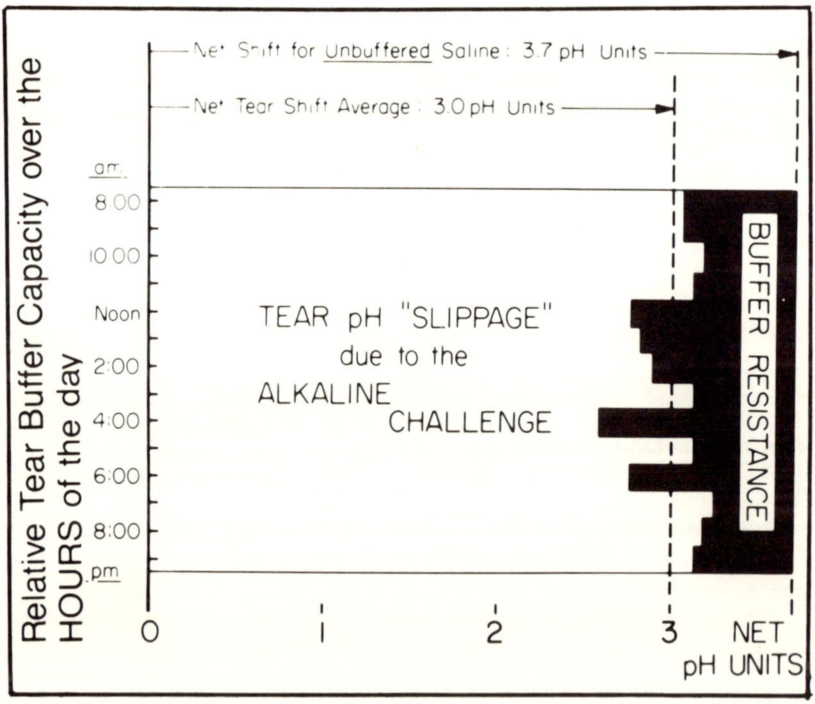

FIGURE 2. The alkaline buffering performance of tear samples collected over the waking hours of the day from a relatively less resistant patient.

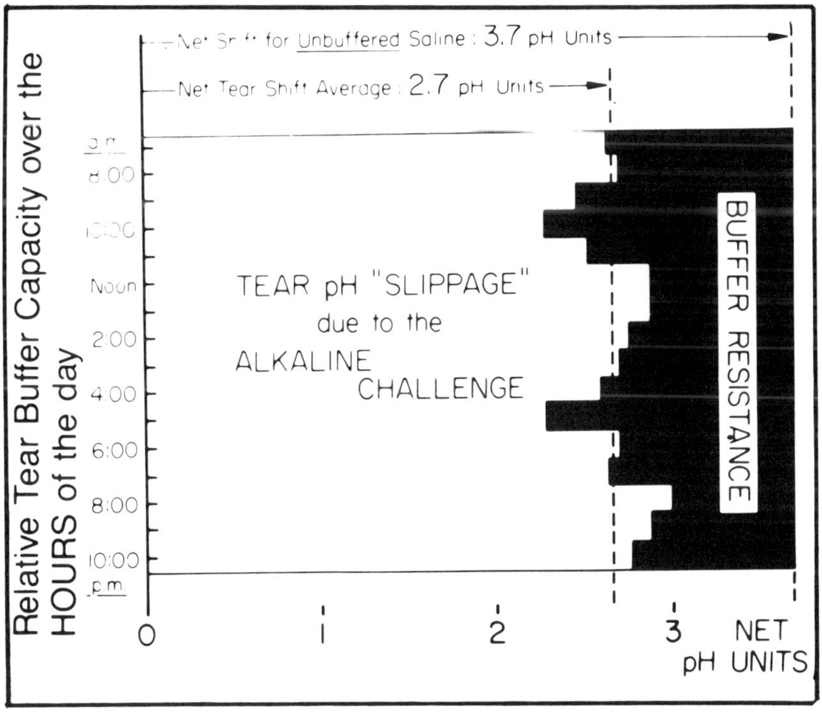

FIGURE 3. The alkaline buffering performance of tear samples collected over the waking hours of the day from a slightly more resistant patient.

hydrogen ions present. If that shift had been 2 pH units to a value of pH 5, there would have been a 100-fold increase, as shown at the right of Figure 1.

The pH unit, then, is a manageable shorthand to describe the immense increases occurring clinically (toward the acid direction) or dilutions (toward the alkaline direction) of hydrogen ions in the tears. (Such changes are actually logarithmic within the common scaling used, where $pH = -\log H^+$.)

The Alkaline "Stress Test"

Cells have limits to their pH tolerance. How well, then, are the tears able to resist extreme changes? We might explore the alkaline part of the spectrum by adding concentrated sodium hydroxide to see how well human tears are able to resist such a severe challenge. Thus, a 1 mm^3 volume of 0.1 NaOH was added to each 10 mm^3 tear sample.

When such an alkaline dose is added to unbuffered saline, that solution is shifted by nearly 4 pH units, as shown in Figure 2. However, tear samples given that same challenge were found to shift not quite as far, thus demonstrating some resistance or buffering capacity.[6] This facility varies throughout the day. It varies most in the generally less resistant patient (shown in Figure 2), but usually somewhat less, as in the slightly more resistant patient (in Figure 3).

"Recruiting" the Resistance

Although the buffering capacity of tears is limited, some factors apparently protect against disturbances of normal pH. What are they?

The best candidates seem to be certain species of proteins, as well as phosphate and ammonium components. Also, the bicarbonate system of the tears neutralizes the acid-producing effects of carbon dioxide as it exits from the cornea, thus assisting also with the maintenance of a pH status quo.[7]

Many clinical subtleties of tear pH and buffering capacity just now are emerging, but they do appear to be interlinked with such wide-reaching phenomena as ocular discomfort, reaction to infection, lysozyme efficiency, gel-lens water balance and oxygen transmissivity, to cite just a few examples. With progressing insight into these mechanisms, however, the practitioner should be better able to predict and manage many of the fitting problems that are chronically resistant to us today.

References

1. Carney, L.G., Hill, R.M., Tear pH and the hard (PMMA) contact lens patient. *Intern. Contact Lens Clinic*, 3(1): 27-30, 1976.
2. Hill, R.M., Carney, L.G., Tear pH and the soft contact lens patient. *Intern. Contact Lens Clinic*, 4(3):71-76, 1977.
3. Moses, R.A., *Adler's Physiology of the Eye*. St. Louis: C.V. Mosby Co., 1975, p. 22.
4. Bitonte, J.L., Keates, R.H., *Symposium on the Flexible Lens*. St. Louis: C.V. Mosby Co., 1972, p. 216.
5. Carney, L.G., Hill, R.M., Human tear pH: Diurnal variations. *Arch. Ophthal.*, 94:821, 1976.
6. Carney, L.G., Hill, R.M., Human tear buffering capacity. *Arch. Ophthal.*, 54:821-824, 1976.
7. Fatt, I., Hill, R.M., Takahashi, G.H., Carbon dioxide efflux from the human cornea, in vivo. *Nature*, 203:728, 1964.

Chapter Three

Escaping the Sting

Certainly a prescription form as comfort-oriented as a hydrophilic contact lens can leave the patient and practitioner in a state of surprise when that all-important first insertion causes a nearly instant stinging or burning sensation. A close inspection of the lens may provide no hint of the problem. Since it had not yet "settled" on the eye, it seems premature to suspect the refinement of fit. Could it be that some kind of subtle infiltration may have occurred when the lens was capped in its vial?

The Outer Fringes

Perhaps the boldest clue to the problem comes from the acidity measurements done by Carney[1] on the unbuffered saline from a group of six previously unopened lens vials (i.e., provided with the original caps from the manufacturing laboratory). The one special characteristic of all the lenses in this group, however, was that they had prescription characteristics that placed them at the outer fringes of the useful fitting range. Each lens had spent a minimum of one year on the "inactive shelf."

A pH check revealed that every one of the six vials contained saline with acidity in the low 5 range (average 5.2). While the pH discomfort threshold varies considerably from patient to patient, this level falls well below the 6.6 threshold that has been cited for the average patient.[2]

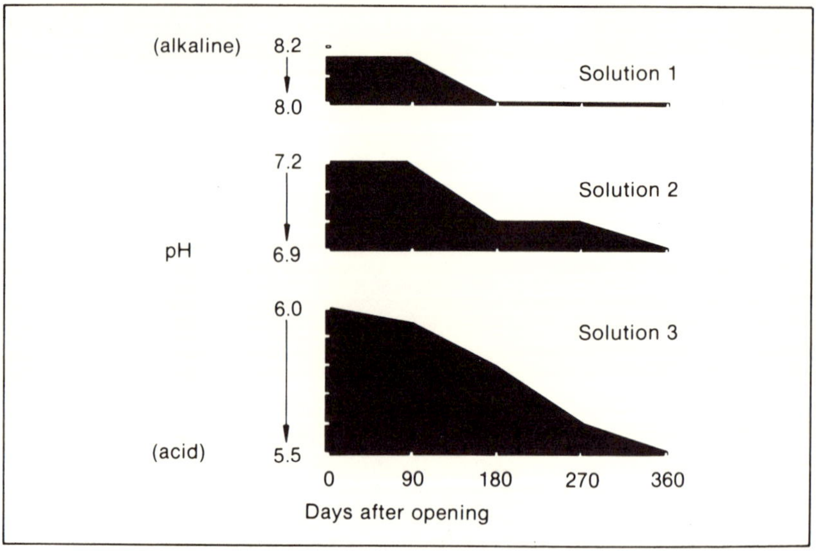

FIGURE 1. The acidward drifts of three different ophthalmic solutions with age. Solution 1 was the most strongly buffered and Solution 3 the least.

When new lenses were checked, however, their saline pH's averaged about 7.3, which is very close to the mildly alkaline level of tears, 7.4.[3] A possible explanation is a gradual permeation of carbon dioxide into the vial through its silicone stopper, causing the saline pH to fall. This is not surprising because certain silicones are known to pass carbon dioxide as well as or even better than oxygen.[4,5]

Vintage Solutions

The "acid lens," due to its saline bath, may be one explanation for the sting, but other possibilities include the vintage lens care solution. In 1973, Young noticed that ophthalmic solutions were in most cases subject to some acidward drift when observed over a long period of time.[6] Figure 1 shows the evolutions of three of the 19 solutions monitored over a one-year period.

The differences in drift were predictable from the degree to which they were buffered, with Solution 1 being the strongest and Solution 3 the most weakly buffered. Although Young concentrated on only hard lens solutions, the results suggest that a careful watch should be maintained on soft lens (and noncontact lens) ophthalmic solutions as well.

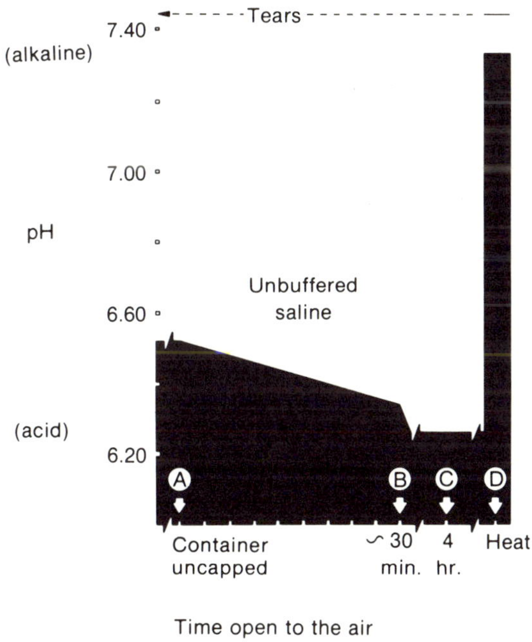

FIGURE 2. the acidward drift of newly constituted saline from the time of first exposure to the air (A), through continual durations of 30 minutes (B), and 4 hours (C). The effectiveness of heating is shown (D) as a means of restoring the pH of that solution back nearly to the level of tears.

Tracking the Descent

Not all solutions take weeks or months to make their acidward descent, however. As noted by Carney,[1] one at least needs only a few hours to show a readily measureable slide—common air-exposed unbuffered saline.

At point A in Figure 2, double-distilled, demineralized water for the constitution of saline was poured from a newly opened container and was found even at that time to have a pH down in the mid-six range (versus 7.0 as neutrality). But even as this newly mixed saline (an unbuffered salt tablet now added) was allowed to stand open to air, enough carbon dioxide was dissolving into it from the atmosphere that 30 minutes later at point B, a further drop of pH was evident, and by point C four hours after mixing, a still greater drop had occurred.

Cures and Concessions

Unlike the very obligatory "concession" of discarding an overaged solution no matter what volume is left, there is a very effective redeeming maneuver where unbuffered saline is concerned. It works for both the capped lens vial and the open solution alike. The answer is *heat*.

As shown in Figure 2, once an unbuffered open saline solution is warmed (even short of boiling), it becomes sufficiently degassed (i.e., the carbon dioxide is driven off) that the pH value rises nearly to the level of tears. The same effect occurs for the unbuffered saline in capped vials, since carbon dioxide can exit back out the same way it originally came in, i.e., through the silicone stopper.[1] In this way heat, followed by rapid use (in the open saline instance), or the routine equivalent of "asceptisizing" for the capped vial case, can become an effective cure for "the sting."

One other method of avoiding "the sting" on a longer range basis is to add a very small amount of sodium bicarbonate to saline to buffer it against such acid descents (written communication from Dr. N.J. Bailey, 1975).

References

1. Carney, L.G., Hill, R.M., Other hydrophilic lens environments: pH. *Amer. J. Optom. and Physiol. Optics*, 53:456-458, 1976.
2. Moses, R.A., ed., *Adler's Physiology of the Eye*, ed. 5. St. Louis: C.V. Mosby, 1970, p. 21.
3. Carney, L.G., Hill, R.M., Human tear pH. *Arch. Ophthal.*, 54:821-824, 1976.
4. Becker, W.E., Corneal Contact Lens Fabricated from Transparent Silicone Rubber, filed June 29, 1962 (3, 228, 741). *U.S. Patent Office Official Gazette*, Jan. 11, 1966, p. 609.
5. Hill, R.M., Cuklanz, H., Oxygen transmissivity of membranes in contact with the cornea. *Brit. J. Physiol. Optics*, 24:206-216, 1967.
6. Young, W.H., Hill, R.M., Ophthalmic solutions. *J. Amer. Optom. Assoc.*, 44:263-270, 1973.

Chapter Four

Aging Ophthalmic Solutions

Until the seal is broken, the expiration date on a solution bottle should give the patient reasonable assurance that the ingredients and the amounts given on the label are indeed those contained inside.* Immediately on opening, however, those contents will proceed to change at some rate (depending on air exposure, time, temperature, mechanical agitation, what might be drawn back inside, etc.) toward new balances with the environment. In this process, desirable properties (e.g., germicidal) may be diminished, while undesirable properties (e.g., increased acidity) may be increased.

But, how rapidly do such changes take place, and what might be the clinical consequences?

The Trends with Time

To explore these questions, a large collection of contact lens solutions was assembled (over a dozen and a half) for the examination of a number of their properties on first opening and then at the end of three-month intervals until one year had elapsed.[2]

*There are, in fact, a few substances which may be lost (or gained) through certain container materials over long periods. Container specifications for minimizing such transfer are given in *The Pharmacopeia of the U.S.A.*[1]

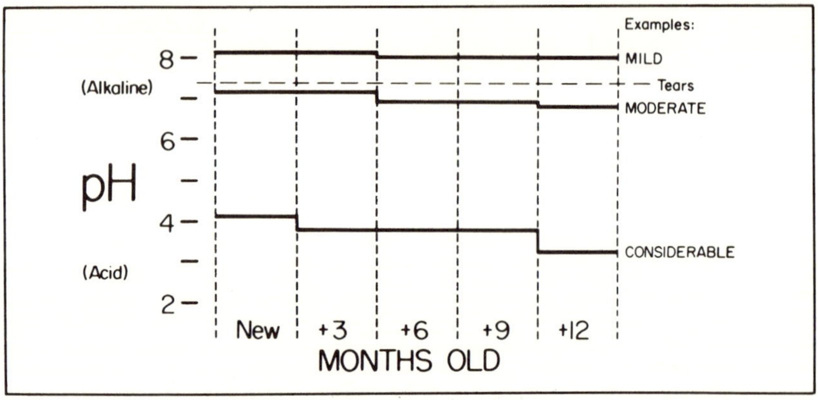

FIGURE 1. Changes of pH over a one-year period after being opened, of three contact lens solutions representative of the mild, moderate, and considerable degrees of change observed.

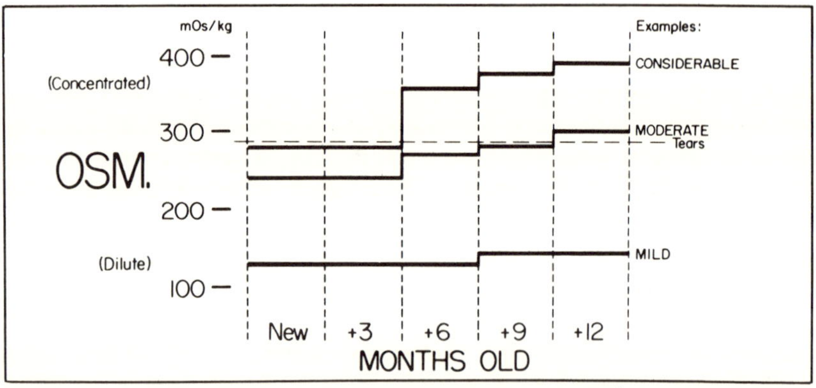

FIGURE 2. Changes of osmotic pressure over a one-year period after being opened, of three contact lens solutions representative of the mild, moderate, and considerable degrees of change observed.

Figure 1 summarizes the spectrum of findings for pH (i.e., alkalinity and acidity) with the progressive histories of three of these solutions which exhibited *mild, moderate,* and *considerable* changes, respectively, with time. Similarly, Figures 2 and 3 show progressive histories for further members of this collection in relation to their osmotic and surface tension properties, respectively.

Clinical Consequences

(1) Every one of the solutions in this survey, although stored at room temperature and capped (being opened only for the five examinations),

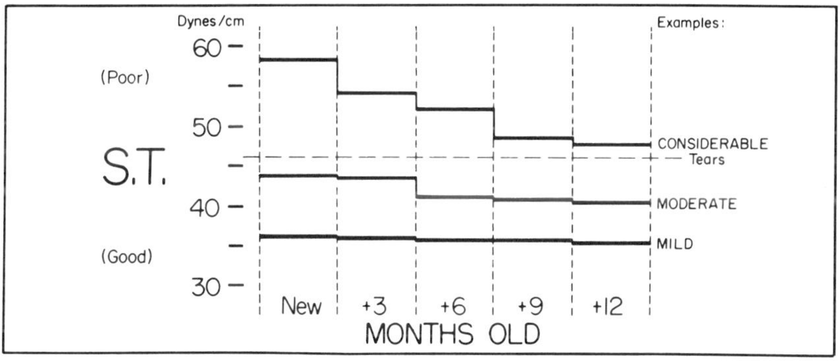

FIGURE 3. Changes in surface tension (ST) over a one-year period after being opened, of three contract lens solutions representative of the mild, moderate, and considerable degrees of change observed.

did show an *acid drift* of pH. This effect may have been in part due to a gradual accumulation of dissolved carbon dioxide. Those whose intial pH values were nearest to tear pH were often the most heavily buffered and changed the least with time. If not adequately rinsed from a lens previous to insertion, those solutions which reached sufficient acid levels could be responsible for an initial discomfort in some patients.[3,4]

(2) The osmotic pressure of every solution *increased*. While evaporation of the aqueous vehicle very likely contributed to this effect, the considerable variability found among solutions suggests that changes (perhaps the breakdown) among the other ingredients have been a factor as well. If sufficiently concentrated (hypertonic) levels are reached, a patient may report complaints of stinging.

(3) Most interesting perhaps was that the surface tensions of all of these solutions *decreased* with time. This may have been due to a concentration of wetting agent ingredients as evaporation of the water vehicle progressed.

The resulting clinical effect would then be one of *increased* wettability.

Risks and Precautions

Although aging did enhance the wetting property of these solutions, that outcome can in no way justify the continued usage of an old ophthalmic solution. Most risky would be the assumption that those minimal levels of germicide present in such containers could still be acting effectively over any extended unsealed period. Certainly those other chemical imbalances described above may too, in their extremes, cause adverse tissue reactions and discomfort.

While perhaps not the most economically attractive, the safest measures to take on behalf of your patient to avoid the aging solution problem are: (1) to encourage from the onset the use of small (limited duration) containers, and (2) to *immediately* discourage any proneness of the patients to refill such containers themselves—a practice rife with contamination potential.

References

1. *The Pharmacopeia of the U.S.A.* 18th Revision, 4630 Montgomery Avenue, Bethesda, Md. 20014, 1970, p. 798.
2. Young, W.H., Hill, R.M., Ophthalmic Solutions. Parts I, II, and III. *J. Amer. Optom. Assn.*, 44:263-270, 1973.
3. Mosses, R.A. (ed.), *Adler's Physiology of the Eye*, 5th ed. St. Louis: C.V. Mosby Co., 1970, p. 21.
4. Davson, H. (ed.), *The Eye Vol. 1*, 2nd ed. New York: Academic Press, 1969, p. 543.

Chapter Five

How Wet Are Your Patients' Tears?

Even in this age of pharmaceutical progress, with its vast array of ophthalmic products, the hard lens patient with chronic wettability problems still persists in many practices today.

Certainly his continued presence raises some vintage questions. Just how different is he in his tear quality from the normal patient? Could he have been spotted at the outset? And, does the erratic nature of his complaints ("some times are surely worse than others") mean that we may be dealing with a "moving target," i.e., an ever changing condition?

How Different?

The easiest way to compare tears from different patients is to see how well they wet onto a standard surface. Because rubber is so difficult to wet, tears will stand in drops very well on such a surface, so that significant differences between a patient's tears and a water drop or another patient's tears can be fairly apparent.

An example is shown in Figure 1 where tears collected from two different patients were placed down on a clean flat silicone rubber surface for comparison. Even without formal measurements, the much better wetting capacity of Patient B's tears (i.e., the much flatter disposition of the drop on the surface) is readily evident.

But how about the next two dozen or so patients to walk into your

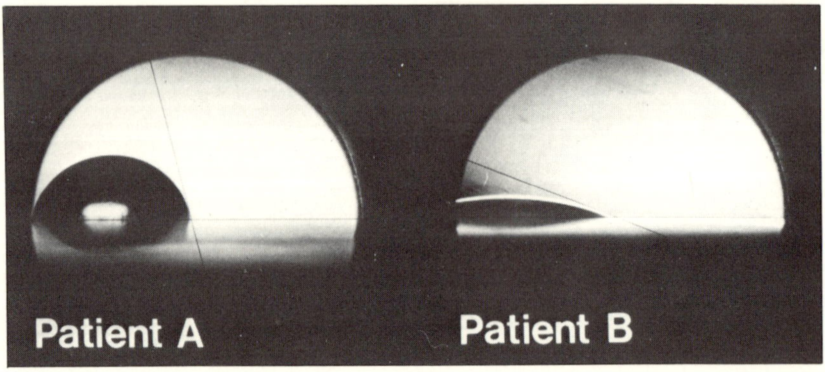

FIGURE 1. The comparative wettability of tears from two different patients.

office—how different will they be? A hint can be gotten from the group of patients represented in Figure 2. In this case their tears were placed down onto an un-prewetted flat PMMA (i.e., conventional hard lens plastic) surface. Although tears from the average patient here had a wetting angle of 52 degrees, some patients had tears which were much more wettable to this plastic surface (angles down to 42 degrees), while others had tears with much poorer wettability (angles up to 60 degrees).

Can the Problem Patient Be Spotted in Advance?

Although tear assessment is still a relatively new clinical procedure, we are far from helpless in such matters. Possibly, the most logical start would be to look for obvious deficiencies in tear wettability by the technique shown in Figure 1. Normal (nonirritating) tears should be collected by allowing a tiny capillary tube (e.g., a 25 lambda standard blood capillary) placed gently under the lower lid to passively fill to about two-third's capacity. These tears can then be placed onto a polished, flat PMMA or rubber surface for viewing (with your slit lamp microscope, for example, or with a loupe). A water drop of the same size can be used as a comparison. Normal tears should lay considerably flatter onto such surface than will water.

Using a very clean standard surface, avoiding evaporation by minimizing inspection time and using about the same size drop volume each time will sharpen your technique.

But Are We Trying to Hit a "Moving Target"?

The erratic nature of wettability complaints suggests that we may be dealing with a continually changing condition. And certainly the findings

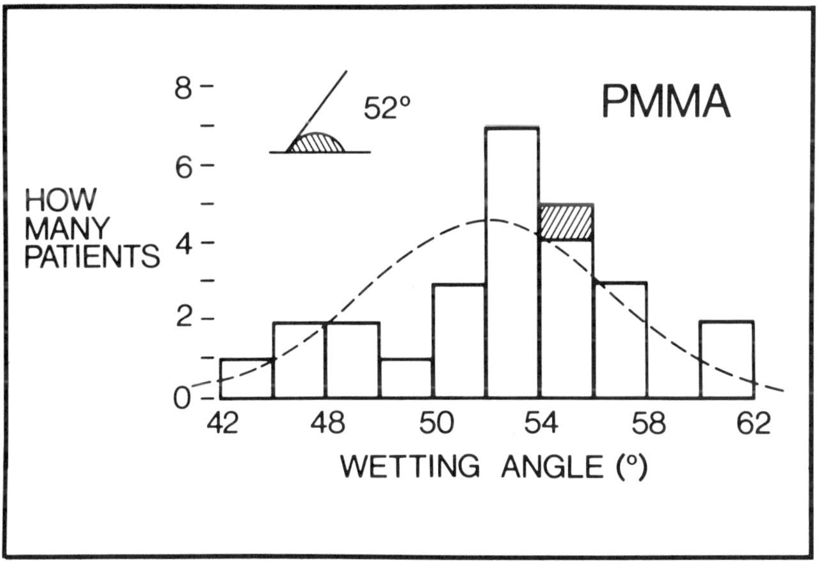

FIGURE 2. Wettability of tears from a small population of patients, on an un-prewetted PMMA (conventional contact lens plastic) surface. The shaded block *represents a patient more closely examined in Figure 3.*

in Figure 3 would seem to support such a suspicion. The 28 tear samples shown there are from one patient, but were collected at different hours and over several days. White her average tear wetting angle on PMMA was 55 degrees (her position in Figure 2 is indicated by the shaded block), the odds appear that her tears will be more wettable (lower angles) in the early morning than late at night.

How Then Is Poor Wettability Managed?

The ultimate answer to this question is always, of course, a highly individual one, one which weighs patient tolerance and motivation, the persistence and severity of the problem and the effectiveness of relief measures (e.g., more frequent removal and re-wetting, rotation of solutions to avoid hypersensitivity, humidifying the environment, etc.). These would be among the most fundamental guidelines to follow:

(1) To question a contact lens candidate carefully at the outset about dry eye signs and symptoms, as well as past contact lens failures.

(2) In cases where the history suggests potential wetting problems, then a direct assessment of tear wettability by some method such as described here would seem merited. If poor wettability is verified, such evidence offers one more tangible basis on which your "proceed or stop" decision can then be made.

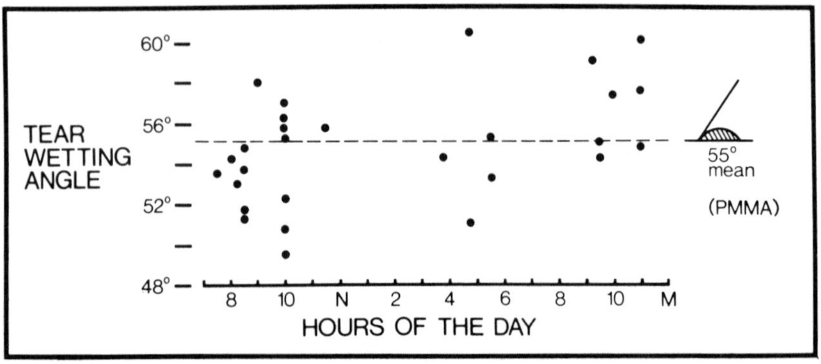

FIGURE 3. Differences in wettability on PMMA plastic of one patient's tears which were collected at various hours over a period of several days. (The shaded block *in Figure 2 represents this patient's position in that population.)*

(3) In instances where a patient has developed wetting problems some time after being fitted, certainly a diligent attempt should be made to isolate any aggravating factors (e.g., a particular environment or time of day) and then to maneuver around them wherever possible.

There is continued hope as well that with time even more effective wetting solutions will evolve, and that the technology of making hydrophilic hard lens plastics will continue to develop. Until then, however, the most expeditious approach to chronic wettability problems still remains to effectively screen those patients out as contact lens candidates at the earliest time possible.

Suggested Reading

Holly, F.J., and M.M. Lemp, The precorneal tear film and dry eye syndromes, in *International Ophthalmology Clinics*. Vol. 13, No. 1. Boston: Little, Brown, 1973.

Chapter Six

Osmotic Vulnerability

Of the many characteristics of tears, their salt content is perhaps the single most critical. While a little extra salt (hypertonicity) can be well tolerated by the cornea, too little salt (hypotonicity) commonly results in the swift and undesirable effect of edema.

But do all patients have the *same osmotic margin of safety*, i.e., are some patients' tears naturally less "salty" than others? And how consistent is a patient's "safety margin" throughout the day? If it varies, when are those critical times?

Is Saline Good Enough?

In the past, saline (0.90 percent NaCl solution) has often been taken as an osmotic benchmark against which body fluids are gauged, but there is evidence now in the case of the cornea that even normal saline may not be quite salty enough to prevent edema. A more effective minimum level of saline might be the equivalent of a 0.93 percent NaCl solution.[1]

Hour by Hour

In exploring the questions asked in the second paragraph, we could include the 0.93 percent NaCl level as a kind of *edema threshold*, as shown in Figure 1. In this format we will be able to trace the osmotic level of a patient's tears throughout the day.

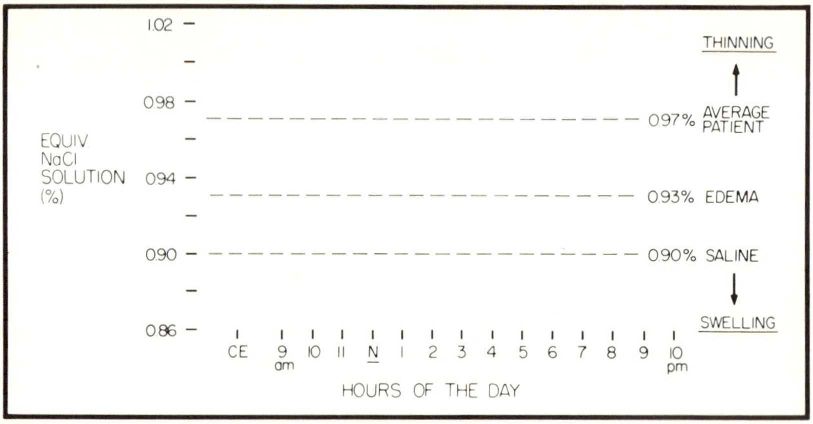

FIGURE 1. A graphical format for monitoring changes in a patient's tear osmotic pressure throughout the day. Several reference levels, including the threshold for corneal edema, are included.

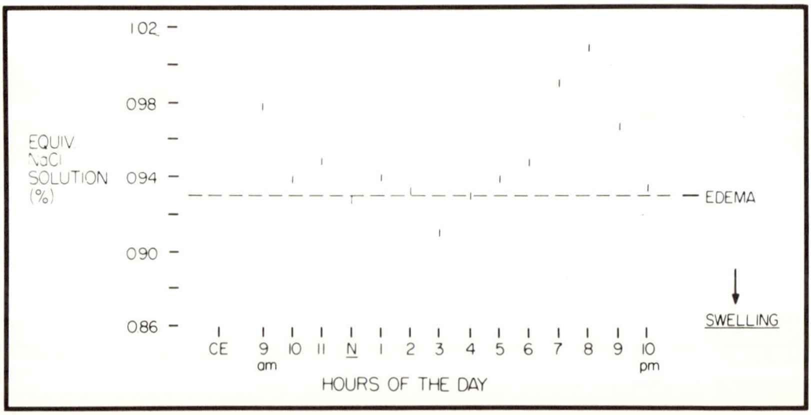

FIGURE 2. Tear osmotic pressure levels recorded for a patient throughout one waking day.

We know from previous studies,[2] that the tears of an average patient are equivalent to about the 0.97 percent NaCl solution level; therefore, the particular corneal thickness associated with that osmotic level might be taken as the clinically normal one for an eye. So again, as indicated in the Figure 1 format, as the salt level falls the cornea will be prone to swell, and as the salt level rises, the cornea will tend to thin.

In Figure 2, the hour-by-hour osmotic levels for one contact lens candidate (prefitted) have been traced on this format. It is the first day of five that was monitored for this patient from waking until retiring. Most

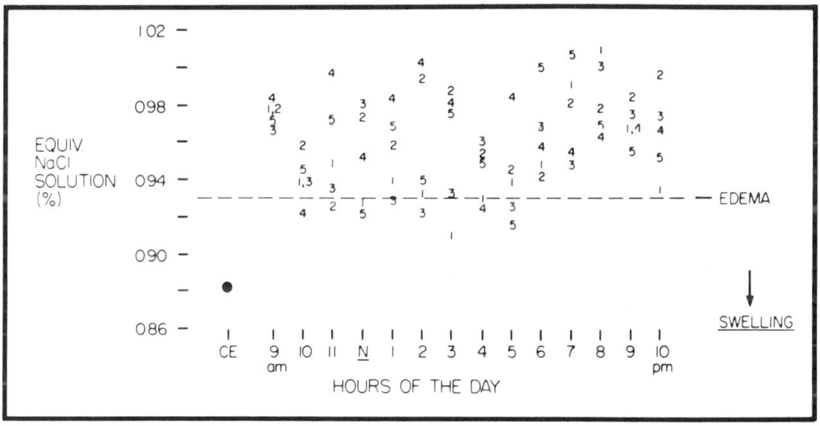

FIGURE 3. Tear osmotic pressure levels recorded for the same patient as in Figure 2, but with findings for four additional days as well. The filled point is a population average of tear osmotic pressures found immediately on awakening, i.e., after prolonged lid closure.

readily evident here, of course, is the relative instability that occurred through that day.

The Critical Points

But is such instability exceptional? Not really. In fact, it appears to be the rule rather than the exception, as shown in Figure 3. Clinically, of course, the most interesting points are those which fall below the edema threshold. In this patient's case about 14 percent of those samples were below this threshold.

The most consistently critical time, however, seems to be associated with the overnight period, when evaporation and its effect of concentrating tear salts is virtually eliminated. The filled point in Figure 3 is the average value found for a population of six patients as they were just awakening (i.e., immediately on first opening of the eye). It would seem, then, that complaints of a blurry world on first awakening may not all be psychological in origin.

Into Perspective

Clinically, then, it appears that:

(1) Since tear osmotic pressure does vary throughout the day, a patient can become periodically more "vulnerable" to corneal edema.

(2) These "vulnerable" times, while somewhat cyclic, do not necessarily occur at the same time every day. In the case of the patient in Figure 3, the end of the day (after 5:00 PM) appears to be a "safer"

period, but this too seems to differ among patients.

(3) Of the six patients monitored in this way so far, first awakening was found to be their most "osmotically vulnerable" time; however, this diluted tear condition was usually corrected well within one hour. For this reason, as well as for oxygen considerations, immediate insertion of contact lenses on arising seems ill-advised.

Perhaps the most immediate clinical value of these observations, however, is to emphasize that patients *are* different in their "osmotic vulnerabilities," and that persistence of corneal edema in a contact lens patient in spite of all measures taken may not be the practitioner's "fault." Rather, the origin of the problem may lie in the fundamental make-up of the patient himself.

References

1. Terry, J.E., The Osmolality of Human Tears, Masters Thesis in Physiological Optics, Ohio State University, Columbus, Ohio, 1975.
2. Terry, J.E., and R.M. Hill, Human tear osmotic pressure: *Arch Ophthal*, 96:120, 1978.

Chapter Seven

Probing the Edema Zone

Edema ranks very probably as the cornea's most universal response to abuse, whether it be due to anoxia, osmotic disturbance, trauma, or disease.[1] What is known of the vital signs of such a lesion (i.e., those indicators of the metabolic activity on which water balance, healing, energy storage, and other processes that maintain normalcy depend)? Could it be that even after the overt indications of edema have disappeared (e.g., visible turgescence and acuity deficits), certain phases of recovery still persist for as long as a day or so?

Probing the Lesion

One such vital sign that can now be monitored is the oxygen uptake within and surrounding an edematous zone.[2] Figure 1 illustrates the oxygen uptake profile across the diameter of a 4mm-round edematous zone. This lesion was produced osmotically be exposing the corneal surface to distilled water contained within a thin-walled cylinder held against the cornea concentric to its optic axis.[3] Measurements made immediately upon removing the distilled-water stimulus showed that the uptake of oxygen was significantly reduced within the zone, at one point to less than three-quarters the normal level.

This reduced flow of oxygen into the cornea may be due in part to the increased resistance (barrier effect) that the edema represents in the path of oxygen-demanding cells deep in the epithelium.

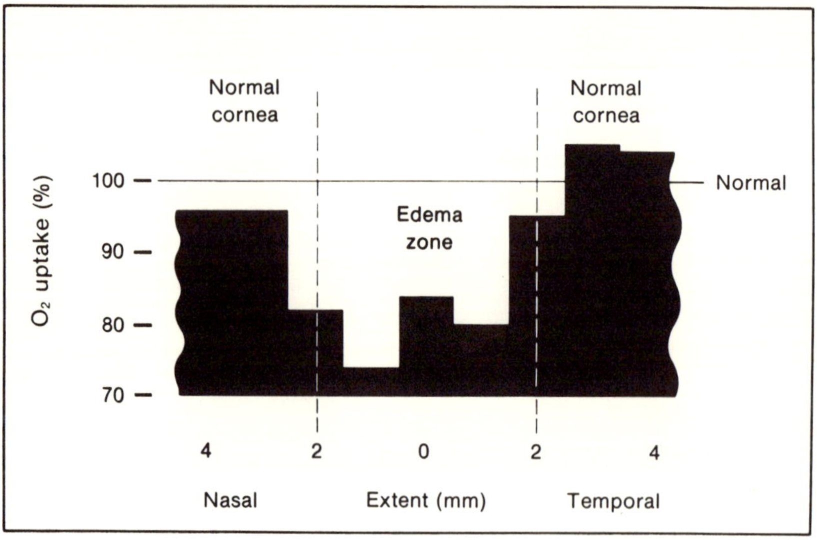

FIGURE 1. The decrease in corneal oxygen uptake across a diameter of a freshly formed edema zone, and for the peripheral region around it.

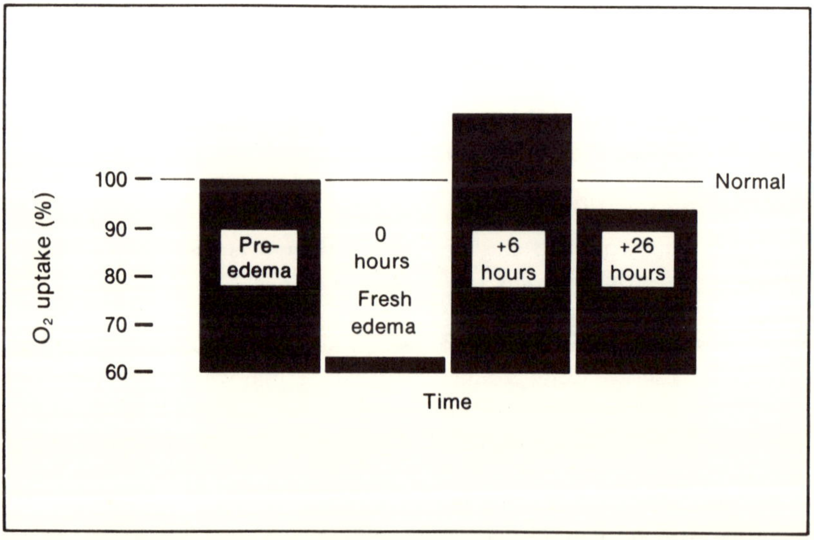

FIGURE 2. The average oxygen uptake for a corneal zone measured previous to edema, for the fresh lesion, six hours later, and 26 hours later.

The Long Return

The question most fundamental to the contact lens fitter would seem to be, When is recovery complete? Although an exact answer will be unique to each case (i.e., dependent on the particular cause, extent, and depth; the interim environment; etc.), Figure 2 indicates that several recovery phases may be passed through, ranging from a stage of "reactive hyperflux," occurring within six hours of return to a normal environment, to a milder but more enduring stage of "reactive hypoflux," at the 26-hour point, poststimulus. In contrast, the clinically detectable indications of this lesion had faded within the first two hours.

It appears then that metabolic vestiges of such an edematous lesion may endure well after physically observable signs have disappeared, being detectable even into the following day. Therefore a little more rather than a little less open-eye recovery time would seem advisable before reintroducing a contact lens to such an eye.

References

1. Mishima, S., Corneal thickness. *Surv. Ophthal.* 13:57, 1968.
2. Hill, R.M., Schoessler, J.P., Epithelial edema: Respiratory characteristics of the lesion. *American J. Optom.* 45:241, 1968.
3. Terry, J.E., Hill, R.M., Human tear osmotic pressure. *Arch. Ophthal.*, 96:120, 1978.

Chapter Eight

Perils of the Pump

Until the *ultimate* contact lens is readily available (that is, one whose properties include a high passage rate of oxygen), the contact lens fitter must continue to fact that irreducible problem of *how to get enough oxygen to the cornea.*

The penalties for failing are well-known of course: *corneal edema* and *reduced vision* (i.e.,"Sattler's veil"). And while some patients do exhibit a remarkable will to live with these problems, no responsible fitter wants to see them continue. Indeed, highest standards of practice dictate termination of wear if an adequate pump can't be established within a reasonable period of time.

Shifting Conditions

Probably most frustrating to the fitter, however, is to have the highly motivated but marginally successful patient return again and again with those classic symptoms of oxygen starvation. What is it that causes such intermittent crises?

One answer might be periodic changes in *lifestyle.* Let's take the patient who lives tolerably with his lenses at sea level, but returns to you from his vacation in Mexico City with tales of irritation. While at home he might be receiving just enough oxygen under his lens to get by (since at sea level there is a full atmosphere at hand to "feed" the pump), Mexico

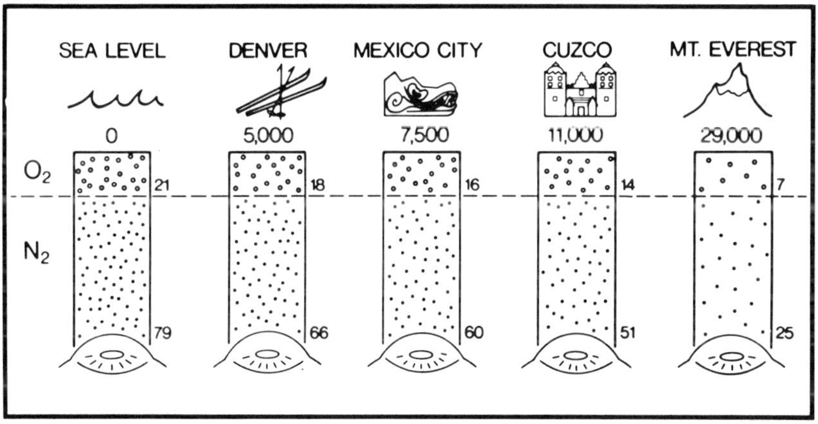

FIGURE 1. A schematic model of the progressive scarcity of oxygen available to the lens pump as a patient travels to higher and higher altitudes.

City is at nearly 8,000 feet altitude where oxygen is somewhat less plentiful.

Figure 1 shows, schematically, those reduced oxygen conditions your patient would be up against. Here, the tear pool under the lens has been blown up so we can see inside. (As an easy model, it shows 21 oxygens inside at sea level and the rest as nitrogen.) But look what happens to our traveling patient as he "fills" his pump in Denver or Mexico City or in the Peruvean Andes (Cuzco), or (for the ultimate explorer) Mt. Everest, the world's highest land point. The higher he goes, the fewer oxygens his pump will pull in with each blink—and ultimately the cornea will begin to suffer.

A Triple Threat

But of course your patient's chronic pump problems are rarely as singular and clearcut as this. They are most often the result of several conditions. Just one example might be the synchronous occurrence of fatigue (resulting in slowed blink rate), an increase in tear thickness (due to dryness of the atmosphere), and perhaps an altitude change as described above.

Reserves and Recourses

But what to do clinically? The most rational approach lies, of course, in identifying the specific causes and eliminating them. But in reality the complexities of patients' lives, their inabilities to accurately describe their problems to you and—most important—their general reluctance to change or give up a part of their lifestyle, makes the "elegant solution" a rare event in contact lens care.

While the eye does have limited reserves and certain physiological strategies for getting over brief rough spots, the continuous compromising of a cornea can't be condoned. Unfortunately, if the patient is not willing to change or if a better design cannot be found, an intermittent wearing schedule (a few hours on; a few hours off) may be considered. Or, at the limit, complete removal (i.e., termination) may be in the best interest of all.

In the interim, however, we can only hope for the rapid arrival of that *ultimate* lens which will solve all such things.

Chapter Nine

The Unblinking Eye

Between blinks the tear pool serves not only as a mechanical support support for the contact lens but also as a kind of savings account to smooth out the oxygen debt of the central cornea.

How much of a reprieve against oxygen starvation does this reservoir represent in the slow or nonblinking eye? Does the shape or size of that tear pool make a detectable difference?

Applying the Impermeable Standard

To answer these questions, a series of spherical concave surfaces of conventional PMMA were placed on a spherical cornea of curvature 47.37DS. After 90 seconds of static (no blink) wearing time, the PMMA surface was removed and the oxygen debt of the central cornea measured. The relative debts associated with eight tear reservoirs formed are summarized in Figure 1 in terms of the dioptric differences between cornea and PMMA surface curvatures, and in Figure 2 in terms of radius differences between the two.*

Three Possibilities

(1) The maximum demand for oxygen by the central cornea after 90

---

*See Reference 1 for calculated fluid volumes and oxygen contents of each reservoir case.

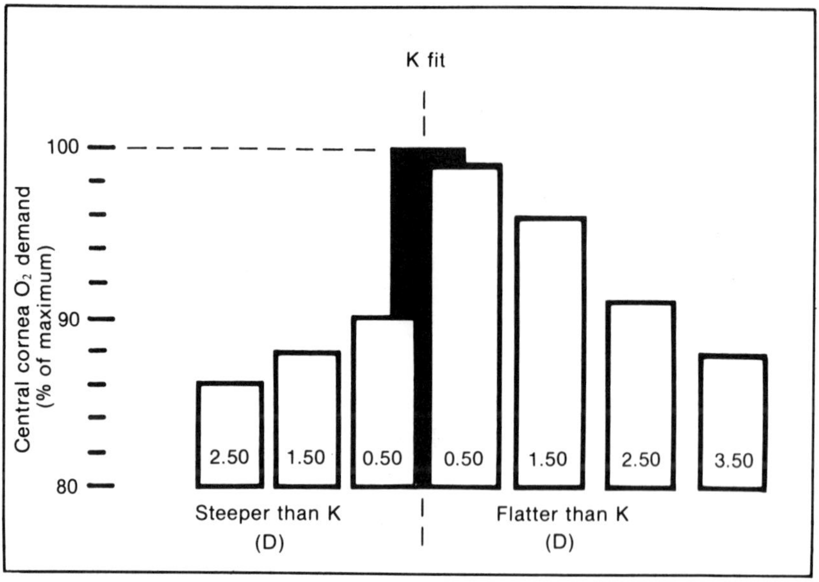

FIGURE 1. Oxygen demands developed by the central cornea following 90 seconds of static (no blink) wear with PMMA fits both steeper and flatter than K expressed in dioptric differences.

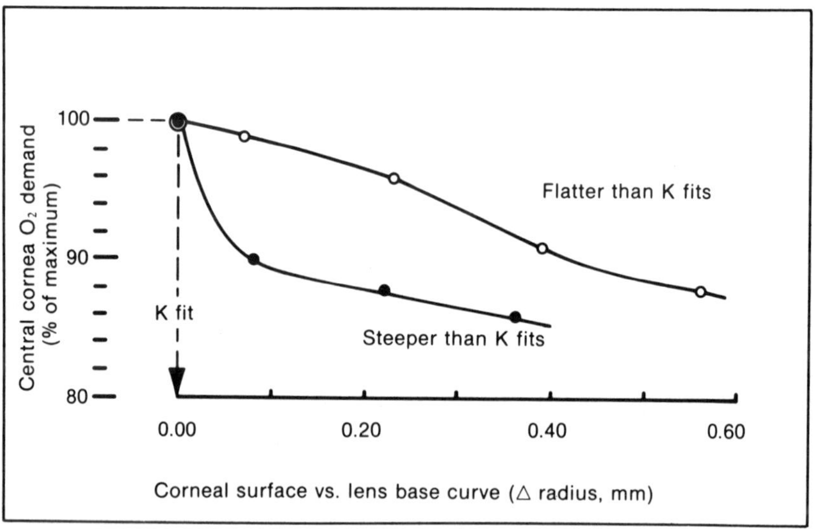

FIGURE 2. Oxygen demands developed by the central cornea following 90 seconds of static (no blink) wear with PMMA fits both steeper and flatter than K expressed in millimeters of Δ radius.

seconds of static (no blink) wearing time was found always to be associated with the on K, or parallel, fit. This condition brought the contained tear volume (and oxygen reserve) to a minimum not only at the central cornea but also out to several millimeters surrounding.

(2) Steep fits did not result in the same severity of debt for that period, since those tear pools formed over the central cornea provided at least short-term assistance. This was evident in even the smallest non-K fit reservoir case.

(3) The degree of oxygen debt was noticeably more sustaining with successively flatter fits, since the PMMA surface remained in closed contact with the central cornea destined to be measured. Relief, then, could come only from the surrounding tear pool as further flattening of the fit allowed it to encroach.

Respiratory Ophthalmometry

The oxygen debts measured above proved sufficiently repeatable—with the K fit consistently producing the maximum—to determine accurately the curvature of the cornea to within 0.37.DS[2] Although it is a tedious and inexpedient way to do that job, the clinical implications of respiratory ophthalmometry, in the cases of slow or non-blinking patients, should not be lost.

REFERENCES

1. Cuklanz, H.D., Hill, R.M., Tear space volumes of spherical and toric cornea-contact lens system. *Amer. J. Optom.*, 45:719-734, 1968.
2. Hill, R.M., Lowther, G.E., Respiratory ophthalmometry. *Amer. J. Optom.*, 45:152-160, 1968.

Chapter Ten

Static . . . and Stagnant

Since a contact lens virtually floats on a thin layer of tears between itself and the cornea, a natural assumption would be that oxygen flows in by that route to meet the needs of the cornea. Under active lid-pump conditions, this is usually so; yet under static conditions, i.e. when the tears themselves are not physically moved, the inevitable outcome with low oxygen permeable lenses is *edema.*

When inflow is reduced then just to diffusion, how near to the edge of a low permeability lens will the epithelium begin to starve for oxygen?

Testing the Corneal Terrain

One approach to that answer would be to directly compare the cornea's demand for oxygen immediately following periods of *no lens* and *lens wear* on the same eye.

Figure 1 shows the oxygen demand at sites 1.5 mm apart across the horizontal diameter of such a cornea.[1] Although slight differences could be detected from site to site, the demand at any given location was never more than 7% from the average for that whole diameter.

But when an oxygen impermeable (conventional PMMA[2]) contact lens, 11 mm in diameter and fitted parallel to the cornea's surface, was allowed to rest unpumped on that eye for just 90 seconds, a marked increase in oxygen demand occurred. Within 0.5 mm of the lens edge it

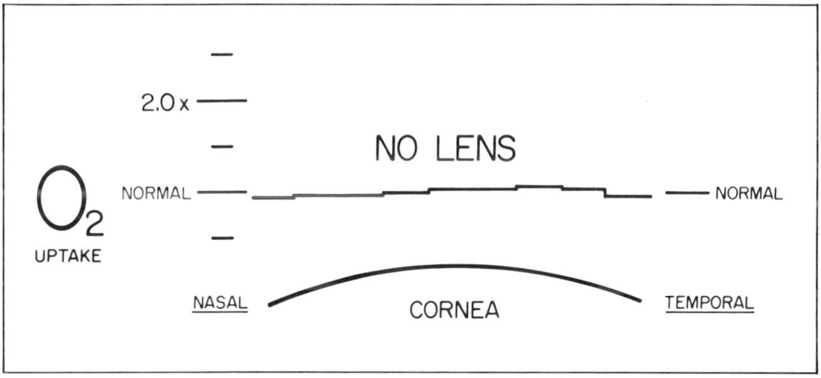

FIGURE 1. Oxygen demands (uptake rates) at 9 sites, 1.5 mm apart across the horizontal diameter of a cornea, which had been freely exposed to the air (no lens).

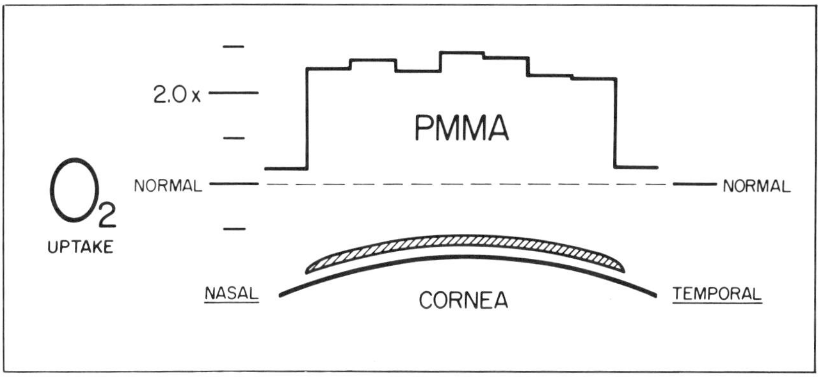

FIGURE 2. Oxygen demands (uptake rates) at 9 sites, 1.5 mm apart across the horizontal diameter of the same cornea as in Figure 1, but after having worn a PMMA contact lens statically for just 90 seconds.

rose to twice the normal rate, and at some sites more internal yet, to nearly 2.5 times normal.

Most interesting however, was the presence of an increased oxygen demand (of some 15% above normal) *just outside* this lens edge, due presumbably to the growing stagnancy of the unstirred tear meniscus between the lens and the corneal surface.

This cornea's response to an unpumped HEMA lens (also cut to an 11 mm diameter and with thicknesses of 0.25 mm at its center and a bit under 0.23 mm at its rolled edge) was very similar as summarized in Figure 2. Considering the very low oxygen permeability of a HEMA lens

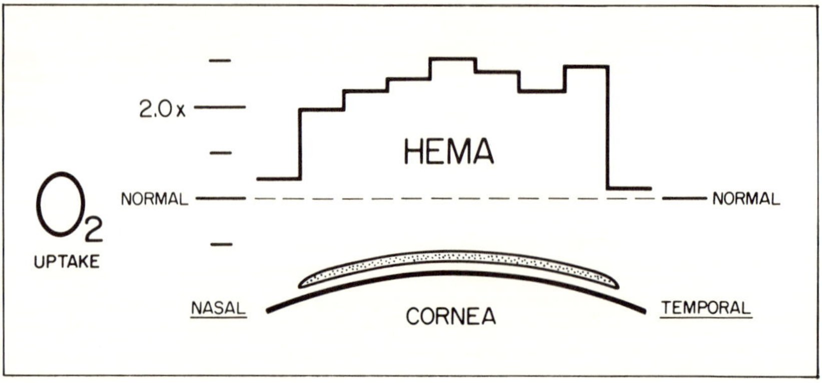

FIGURE 3. Oxygen demands (uptake rates) at 9 sites 1.5 mm apart across the horizontal diameter of the same cornea as in Figure 1, but after having worn a thick HEMA contact lens statically for just 90 seconds.

of those prescription characteristics, the results obtained were not unexpected.[3]

Figment vs Fate

It appears then that the lateral passage of oxygen under the edge of a static, low permeability contact lens is physiologically insignificant, and that common clinical experience with the unpumped lens has been, once again, verified in the laboratory.

But fortunately, of course, there are now several alternatives to that edematous fate, including lenses of high water content or of reduced overall thickness, and those too of the negligible water content families, such of the silicones.[3,4] Even with such promising options, however, the presence of a functioning lid-pump still tends to carry with it a certain measure of comforting clinical assurance.

References

1. Hill, R.M., Effects of hydrophilic plastic lenses on cornea respiration, *Journal. Am. Optom. Assn.* 38:181, 1967.
2. *Physiochemical Properties of Conventional Hard Plastic Contact Lenses.* New York: American National Standards Institute (ANSI Z80.6 - 1976).
3. Hill, R.M. Oxygen permeable contact lenses: How convinced is the cornea? *Intern. Contact Lens Clinic* 4:34, 1977.
4. Benjamin, W.J., and Hill, R.M., Ultra-thins: An oxygen update. *Contact Lens Forum* 4:43, 1979.

Chapter Eleven

Can You Overcome the Oily Lens?

The *oily lens syndrome* will eventually be encountered in virtually every active contact lens practice. Its characteristics commonly include intermittent blurring, greasy lenses, a proneness to deposits, and often conjunctival dry spots.

The Prophylactic Approach

Since the oily lens syndrome is very difficult to manage once it is established, the first (and often the only effective) step is to try to prevent it by a careful screening of all contact lens candidates at the outset.

What are the clues a patient might present? Figures 1 and 2 (representing men and women, respectively) summarize 16 patient histories from a study of tear cholesterol and various clinical factors that might relate to it.[1] For example:

(1) *Blood (serum) cholesterol* — On those occasions when a patient might have this information from a recent medical examination, would it be predictive of the tear level as well? For the most part, no. (Note that those patients with the higher blood levels in the Figures were not consistently those with higher tear levels.) The one exception to this was a rise in both blood and tear cholesterol levels observed in some patients about five hours following a very large cholesterol intake.

(2) *Relative (over- or under-) weight* — As can be seen from the

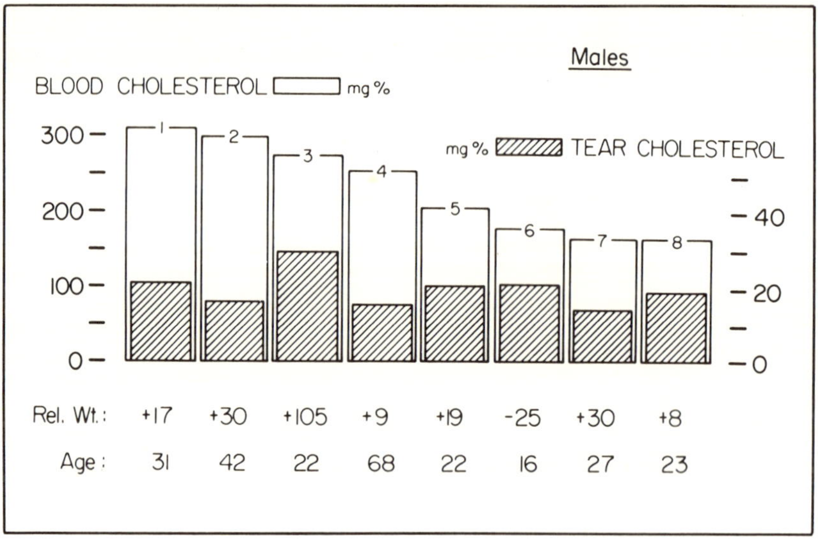

FIGURE 1. The age, relative (over + or under −) weight (lbs.), tear and blood cholesterol histories of eight male patients.

Figures, being over- or underweight related very poorly to either the blood or the tear cholesterol levels of this population.

(3) *Patient age* — Similarly, patient age was a less than satisfactory predictor of tear cholesterol levels.

It appears, then, that three of the most likely predictors one might clinically have chosen are of dubious value; yet at least one procedure may prove both quick and effective for such screening purposes.

Following the logic that it is an adversely "sticky" quality that oily components bring to the tears, a test for tear *viscosity* should serve very appropriately as a prophylactic screener of such problem candidates. Measuring tear viscosity is a procedure usually requiring no more than 15 or 20 seconds and very little instrumentation (a loupe and a penlight can serve). The technique, fully outlined by Schuller, Young, and Hill,[2] is simply to estimate the rate of particle movement in the lower tear prism toward the nasal canthus of the eye and to interpret your observation from a chart scale of five steps.

Clinical Crises

But what if an *oily lens* patient slips through your screening procedure, or, as often happens, you inherit such a contact lens patient complete with this classical history from another practitioner? As a class, they clearly rank among the most difficult problem patients to deal with —

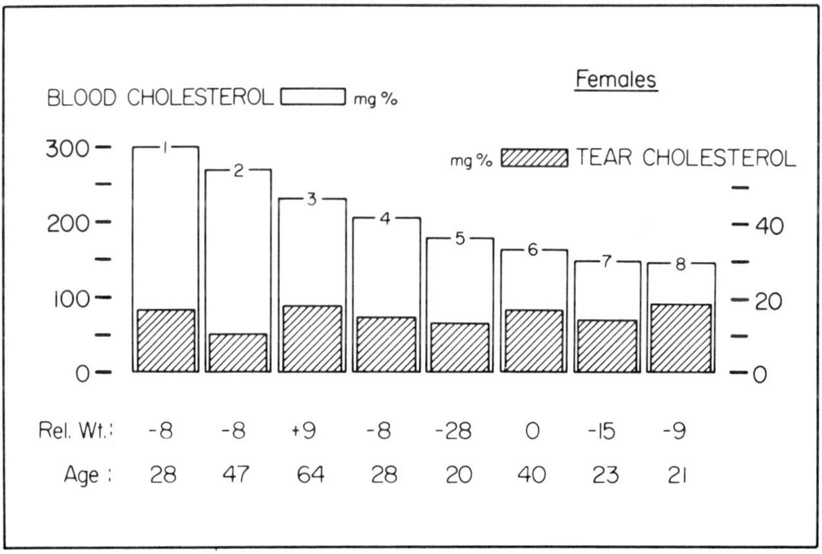

FIGURE 2. The age, relative (over + or under −) weight (lbs.), tear and blood cholesterol histories of eight female patients.

often not because there are no workable solutions, but rather because such solutions may demand a change in lifestyle which the patient is unwilling to comply with (e.g., a long-term low-cholesterol diet).

Some success in managing such cases has been realized, however,[3] so optimism is merited as long as patient motivation and practitioner understanding prevail.

References

1. Hill, R.M., Terry, J.E., Human tear cholesterol levels. *Arch. Ophthal.*, 36:155-160, 1976.
2. Schuller, W., Young, W.H., Hill, R.M., Clinical measurements of the tears: Viscosity. *J. Amer. Optom. Assoc.*, 43:1358-1361, 1972.
3. Young, W.H., Hill, R.M., Cholesterol levels in human tears: Case reports. *J. Amer. Optom. Assoc.*, 45:425-428, 1973.

Chapter Twelve

Fathoming the Postlens Tear Pool

For tens of decades (e.g., Scheiner's observations in 1619) the complexities of the corneal surface have fascinated theorist and fitter alike. Could there be any more geometrically confounding aspect of the contact lens system to deal with?

Yes! What about the nature of the tear pool held between the lens and cornea? Apart from confirming its presence and estimating its depth by fluorescein, what actual volume is captured there between blinks? In tangible units such as cubic millimeters, how much tear flow might be expected around the lens edge per blink?

Bending the Base Curve

The two-sphere model of Cuklanz and Hill,[1] which for simplicity treats both the front of the cornea and the back of the lens as spherical surfaces in gentle contact, can be useful for a first-order exploration of these volume questions.

For example, if we apply the model to a cornea of the most common curvature, 7.8 mm, we find an increase in postlens tear volume with every increasing departure of the lens base curve from that radius, both in the steeper and flatter directions[2] (Figures 1 through 4). The tear pool in the steepening cases assumes (ideally, of course) an increasingly domelike configuration, while in the flattening cases a deeping annulus is formed

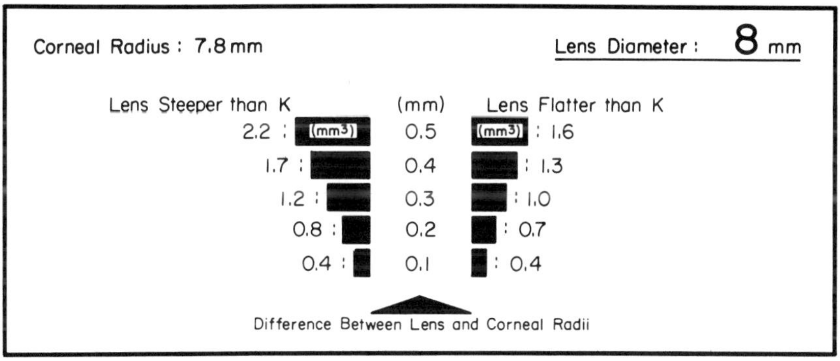

FIGURE 1. Tear volumes expected between spherical lenses of 8 mm diameter (with base curves ranging from 3D steeper to 3D flatter than K) and a cornea of 7.8mm radius (see text).

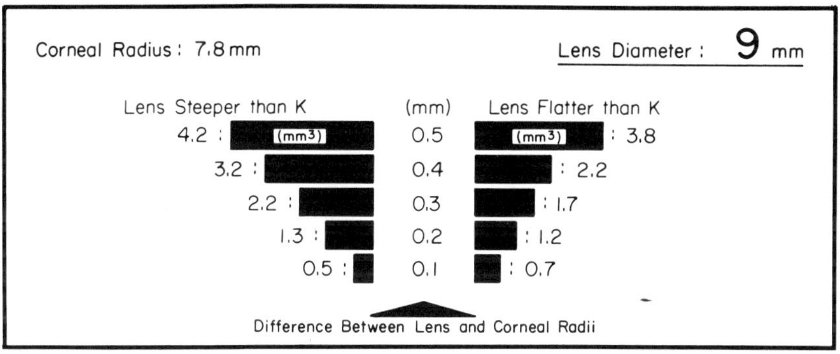

FIGURE 2. Tear volumes expected between spherical lenses of 9 mm diameter (with base curves ranging from 3D steeper to 3D flatter than K) and a cornea of 7.8mm radius (see text).

around a central (optic axis) touch point, just as is viewed with fluorescein.

The powerful effect of lens diameter as a tear volume determinant under the lens is readily evident from the sample series shown here (contrast the 8mm-diameter case in Figure 1 with the 12mm-diameter case in Figure 4). However, it must be realized as well that this model becomes more and more approximate as lens diameter increases, since in practice both lens and corneal surfaces make their greatest departures from sphericity as the limbus is approached. The values for the larger diameters, then, are probably biased due to various combinations of corneal flattening and the incorporation of lens secondary curves.

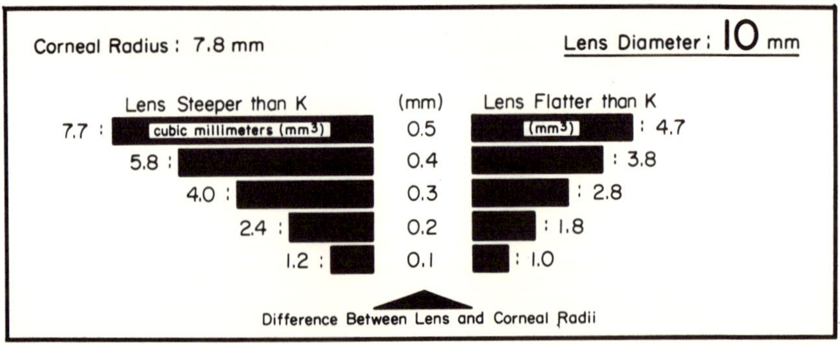

FIGURE 3. Tear volumes expected between spherical lenses of 10mm diameter (with base curves ranging from 3D steeper to 3D flatter than K) and a cornea of 7.8mm radius (see text).

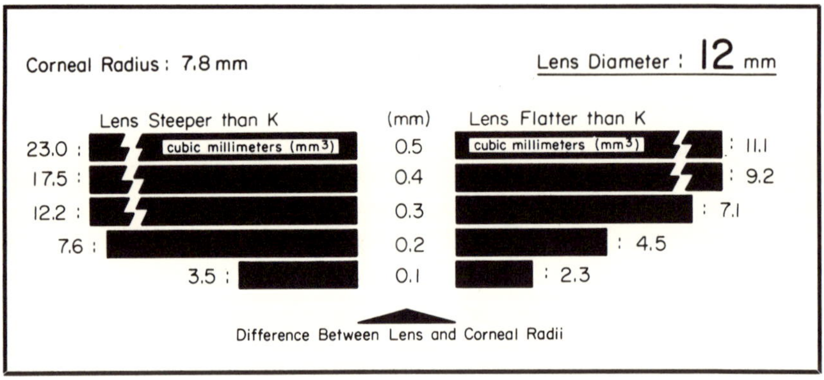

FIGURE 4. Tear volumes expected between spherical lenses of 12mm diameter (with base curves ranging from 3D steeper to 3D flatter than K) and a cornea of 7.8mm radius (see text).

Estimations Versus Expectations

Approximate as this model is, however, it can be relatively useful for comparing actual versus expected tear flow at the lens periphery. One basis for such gauging would be to use the range measured for several tear pumps observed in the laboratory: 10 to 17 percent of the postlens pool volume exchanged per blink. Coupling this exchange range with the calculated value of the total postlens pool volume—available in graphic form for corneas of 6.7 to 8.6 mm radii through four lens diameters—the expected flow per blink can be obtained easily in cubic millimeters for direct clinical comparison at the lens edge.[3]

Although the model described here may be as accurate as clinical measurements now merit, the technology nevertheless exists even today, in the form of advanced photokeratometry and computer processing, for far more individualized and accurate treatment of such design problems. Certainly, with continuing gains in the benefits-to-cost ratio of these methods, even these highly sophisticated methods may come within clinically practical reach in the not-too-distant future.

References

1. Cuklanz, H.D., Hill, R.M., Tear space volumes of spherical and toric cornea-contact lens systems. *Ameri. J. Optom.*, 45:719, 1968.
2. Cuklanz, H.D., Hill, R.M., Tear volumes between contact lens and cornea. *J. Amer. Optom. Assoc.*, 40:264, 1969.
3. Cuklanz, H.D., Hill, R.M., Oxygen requirements of corneal contact lens systems. *Amer. J. Optom.*, 46:228, 1969.

Part II: THE CORNEA

Probing an extraordinary need for oxygen: How it can vary with temperature, lid closure, injury and anesthesia; differences in need among patients, and some local competition.

Chapter Thirteen

The Cornea's Need to "Breathe"

Of all practitioners concerned with the eye, it must surely be the contact lens fitter who is most keenly aware of the cornea's need for oxygen. What was early described as "outer suffocation" and later called "Sattler's veil" (i.e., the signs and symptoms of contact lens induced edema) was directly linked by the 1940s to a chronic shortage of oxygen.[1]

Today, however, the cornea's need for oxygen can be observed even more directly—by looking right under a contact lens as it is "pumped" on the eye. This can be done through a tiny oxygen sensor buried into the lens itself. What is seen as the lens is worn is a series of events, as shown in Figure 1, where the amount of oxygen available to the cornea is registered on the vertical axis and contact lens wearing time is shown on the horizontal axis.[2]

The Critical Blink

Most critical to the cornea's regular supply of oxygen, however, is the blink rate of the patient, a fitting fact long appreciated by the contact lens practitioner. Notice in Figure 1 that when the lens is pumped very rapidly (blink interval of one second), the level of oxygen stays very high, approaching the level of the atmosphere— 21 percent (or 155 mm Hg on the y-axis of the figure). But as the blink rate slows (notice the blink

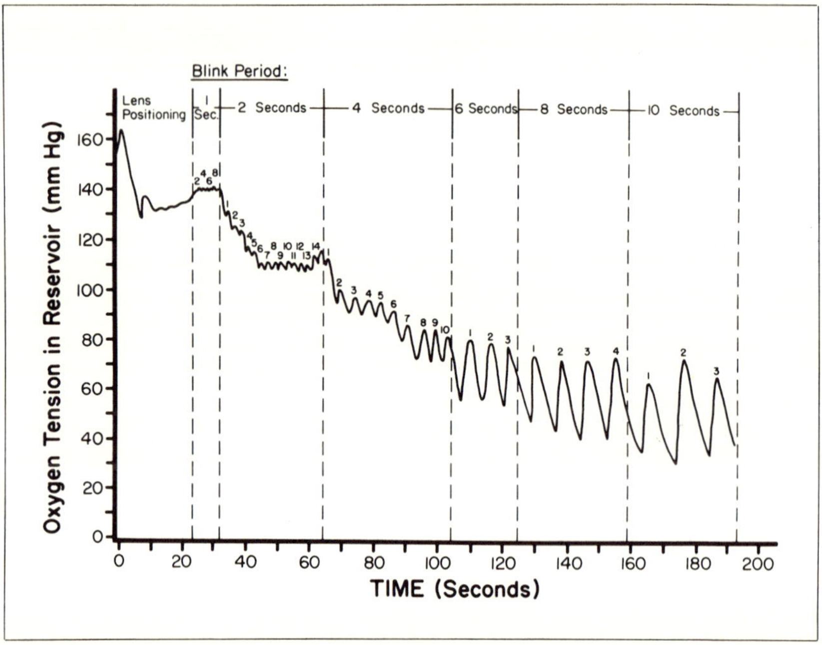

FIGURE 1. Oxygen available to the cornea under a PMMA contact lens at different blink rates. 155 mm Hg is about 21 percent oxygen; i.e., the normal atmosphere. The downstroke of each "sawtooth" is due to the cornea's uptake of oxygen from the tear pool under the lens between blinks; the upstroke reflects the insurge of fresh oxygen with each blink.

intervals of six, eight and ten seconds), the amount of oxygen under the lens falls considerably as well.

How Little Is Enough?

But what is the minimum amount of oxygen on which the cornea can subsist under a contact lens? Here the practitioner has a range of choices from the two-percent level (about 15 mm Hg on the graph) of Polse and Mandell,[3] which results in corneal edema readily demonstrated by pachometry (measuring slitlamp), to the five-percent (about 40 mm Hg) level of Uniacke et al.,[4] below which the energy (glycogen) reserves of the cornea melt away. Or, for a more "natural" criterion, the 7 to 8 percent level (about 60 mm Hg) estimated for the closed eye[5] might be used.

Implications for Hydrophilic Lenses

Certainly the cornea's "thirst" for oxygen will be as great under a hydrophilic contact lens as under a hard one made of PMMA, but, of course, in the case of a hydrophilic lens there is a second oxygen route available; i.e., through the lens itself.

How efficient is the route, however? Using a living eye technique (the "equivalent oxygen method"[6]), most materials readily available today appear to have oxygen passages of 0.5 to 10.0 percent over the common range of center thicknesses used. While even this limited amount is a significant assist, *assurance of a supplementary mechanical pump* (e.g., by a millimeter or two of the lens movement with each blink) must still remain foremost among the fitter's criteria when striving for a best-performance design.

References

1. Dallas, J., Sattler's veil. *Brit. J. of Ophthal.*, 30:607, 1946.
2. Hill, R.M., and J.P. Schoessler, Tear pumps: Reservoir oxygen measured in situ. *J. Am. Optom. Assn.*, 40:1102, 1969.
3. Polse, K. and R.B. Mandell, Critical oxygen tension at the corneal surface. *Arch. Ophthal.*, 84(4):505-508, 1970.
4. Uniacke, C.A., Hill, R.M., Greenberg, M. and S. Seward, Physiological tests for new contact lens materials. *Amer. J. Optom.*, 49(4):329-332, 1972.
5. Fatt, I. and R.D. Freeman, Oxygen tension distributions in the cornea: A re-examination. *Exp. Eye Res.*, 18:357, 1974.
6. Hill, R.M. and W.H. Jeppe, Hydrogels: Is a pump still necessary? *Intern. Contact Lens Clinic*, 2:27, 1976.

Chapter Fourteen

Anoxia: The Ultimate Debt

Among the persistent problems that can plague a contact lens system, a deficient supply of oxygen to the cornea may be the most serious. Previous to this age of many materials, the threat of severe oxygen "starvation" was, of course, considerably greater. It was most classically represented by the "tight lens syndrome" which had just two requirements (1) a material (e.g., PMMA) which transmitted no significant oxygen, and (2) an inadequate pump to move oxygenated tears under the lens.

The results of that combination remain impressive even today, although their occurrence in full spectrum (e.g., edema, reduced visual acuity, cell loss, pain vessel ingrowth) are increasingly rare. The reasons for this favorable trend are at least two: first, a better appreciation for the oxygen needs of the cornea,[1,2] as summarized in Figure 1; and second, a growing number of new materials coming within clinical reach, whose performances[3] are known with regard to the demands indicated in Figure 1.

One Last Look

For little more than nostalgic reasons, then, we might take just one last look at corneal anoxia at its worst—generated here in the most time-proven way, i.e., under a non-pumping, oxygen impermeable contact lens.

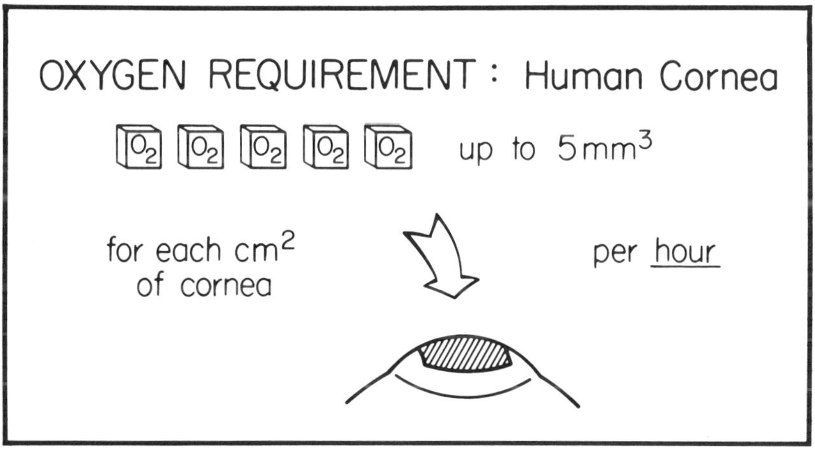

FIGURE 1. Oxygen demand of the human cornea.

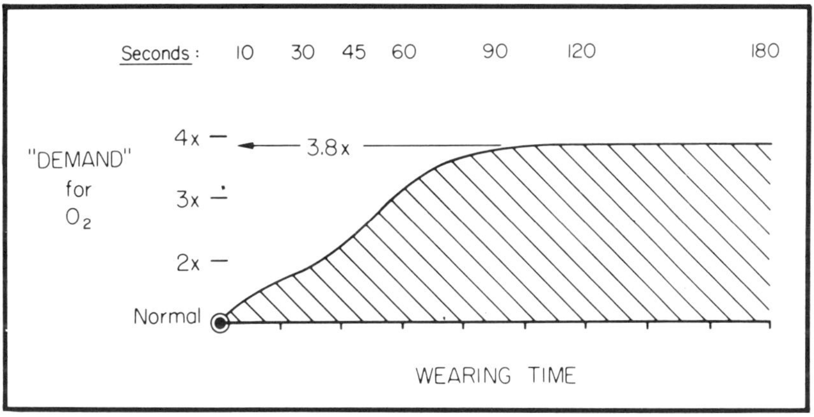

FIGURE 2. Increase in oxygen demand when the cornea is blocked from the atmosphere by an immobile, non-transmitting contact lens.

As summarized in Figure 2, the effect is both swift (reaching maximum by 90 seconds) and severe (an increase in the demand for oxygen of nearly four times normal), and in prolonged status is the exact prerequisite for those several forms of corneal malaise listed earlier.

Emerging Alternatives

Certainly, greater vigilance and improved clinical techniques have greatly reduced the chances of such extreme effects today. But a concurrent, and even more direct solution, to this problem is emerging through those several families of oxygen permeable materials now appearing in lens form.

While silicone, the oldest one to be explored (in this country at least), still remains the best oxygen performer, other groups such as the oxygen permeable hard types are gaining in effectiveness as well. Hydrophilics, too, continue to show promise not only through higher water contents (and other chemical variations) which commonly improve oxygen transfer but also by their successful invasion into the "ultra-thin" domain (i.e., lens center thickness ranging from 0.10mm down to 0.02mm).[4]

Continued improvement in both materials and technique remains especially vital, however, as we progress into the new Age of Extended Wear, most particularly as regards those challenges of the prolonged closed eye (sleep) with its oxygen impoverished environment.[5]

References

1. Hill, R.M. and Fatt, I., Oxygen uptake from a limited volume reservoir by *in vivo* cornea. *Science*, 142:1295, 1963.
2. Juaregui, M.J. and Fatt, I., Estimation of oxygen tension under a contact lens. *Amer. J. Optom.* 48:210, 1971.
3. Refojo, M.F., Contact lenses, in *Encyclopedia of Polymer Science and Technology* Suppl. 1, New York: John Wiley, 1976, p. 195.
4. Hill, R.M., Hydrogel lens design: The thick and thin of it. *Excerpta Medica* (in press, 1977).
5. Hill, R.M., Behind the closed lid: The eye and the contact lens, *Intern. Contact Lens Clinic*, 4(1):68-70, 1977.

Chapter Fifteen

The Cohabitations of a Cornea

Environmentally at least, the cornea lives two markedly different lives. As summarized by Table 1 (p. 60), in the *open eye* case, the corneal temperature and thus its oxygen demand will be down, while the availability of oxygen (i.e., via the atmosphere), the tear salt level (hypertonicity),[1] and the tear pH (alkalinity)[2] will each be at its highest—five physiological "pluses" for deturgescence and transparency. In the *closed eye* case, the opposite trends prevail.

Let us concentrate on the oxygen aspect of the closed eye problem and ask, Just how much oxygen does the cornea get when the lid is closed, and how much more aggravating might the addition of a soft contact lens be to the closed eye?

Three May be a Crowd

As Figure 1 indicates, the lid and cornea alone represent a reasonably compatible combination. The model of Fatt et al. (1974)[3] predicted that the lid, via its palpebral conjunctiva, would provide the cornea with some 7 to 8 percent oxygen (versus 21 percent in air). The measurements of Roscoe and Hill[4] indicate that the cornea may be receiving just under 5 percent by this route. In either case, however, the Polse-Mandell criterion for adequate oxygen (about 1.5 to 2.5 percent) necessary for the

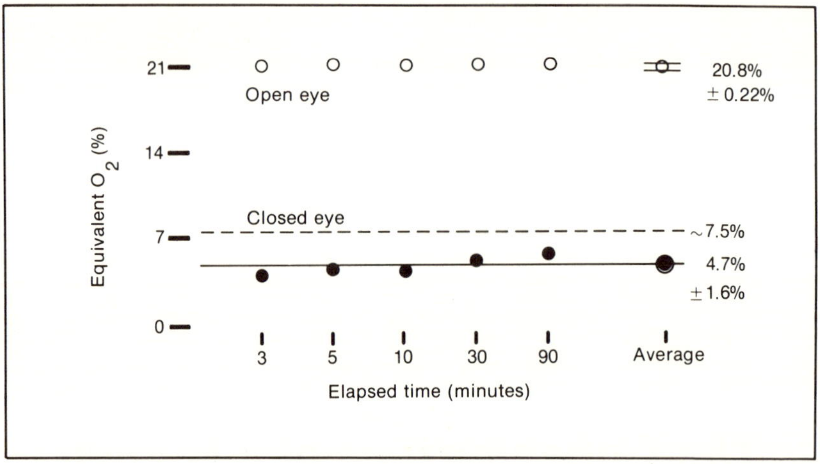

FIGURE 1. Equivalent oxygen responses of the cornea under open eye (open points) and closed eye (closed points) conditions maintained for various periods of time. The dashed horizontal line is a closed eye model estimate,[3] and the solid horizontal line is the average of the measured closed eye points shown here.[4]

prevention of clinically significant swelling[5] has been met some twofold or more.*

The introduction of a contact lens between the lid and cornea can create a significant barrier to the passage of oxygen under certain conditions, even in the case of a silicone material (an experimental form from the Dow-Corning Corporation), as shown in Figure 2. Although when worn on the open eye the silicone lens was virtually undetectable (even at 0.25mm center thickness), under closed eye conditions the cornea responded as if it were receiving about one-half the amount of oxygen it would have got without the lens in place. That level, 2.4 percent, is at the upper boundary of the Polse-Mandell zone.

A cosmetic HEMA lens (Bausch & Lomb Soflens®) of 38.6 percent water content and 0.15mm center thickness, however, was found to fall within the Polse-Mandell zone limits (2.4 percent) under open eye conditions, and it appeared to allow virtually no (physiologically significant) oxygen to reach the cornea under closed eye conditions, as shown in Figure 3.

---

*Lid closure overnight has been noted to cause subclinical levels of cornea edema, possibly as much as 3 to 4 percent, but this is rapidly relieved on reexposure to the atmosphere.[6]

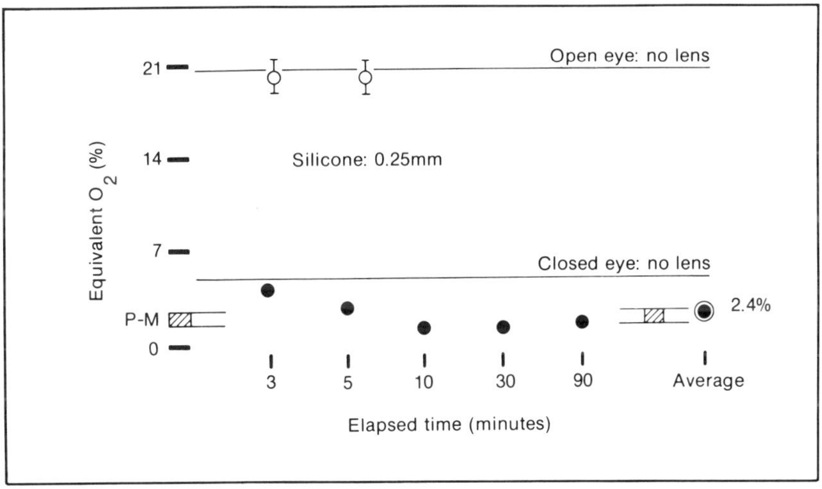

FIGURE 2. Equivalent oxygen responses of the cornea under open eye (open points) and closed eye (closed points) conditions to an experimental silicone lens maintained in place for various periods of time. Open and closed eye corneal responses with no lens are given, as well as Polse-Mandell zone (P-M, brackets) limits.

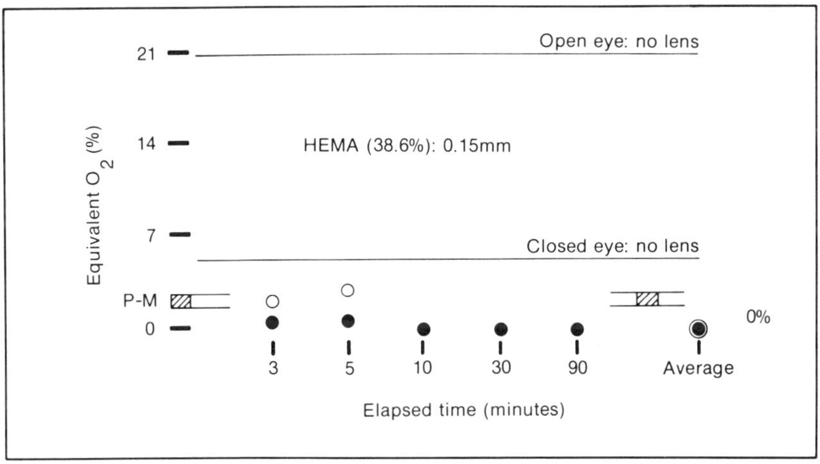

FIGURE 3. Equivalent oxygen responses of the cornea under open eye (open points) and closed eye (closed points) conditions to a HEMA lens of 38.6 percent water content, maintained in place for various periods of time. The open eye and closed eye corneal responses with no lens in place are given, as well as the Polse-Mandell zone (P-M, brackets) limits.

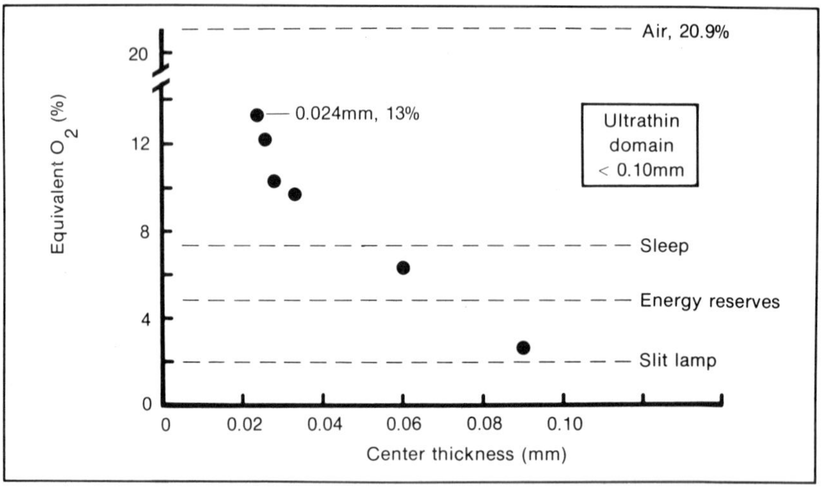

FIGURE 4. The improvement in oxygen passage through a HEMA lens of 38.6 percent water content as center thickness is progressively reduced (toward the left) below 0.10mm (i.e., into the "ultrathin domain").

TABLE 1

A comparison of corneal environments.

Open eye		Closed lid
↓	Temperature	↑
↓	O_2 demand	↑
↑	O_2 supply	↓
↑	Tear salt	↓
↑	Tear pH	↓
5 pluses		5 minuses

"Happiness is a Thin Cornea 'Breathing' Well"

If deturgescence and transparency are to be counted high on the priority list for patient (and practitioner) satisfaction, silicone certainly appears to be a promising clinical prospect. Prolonged wettability and surface build-up control must be well assured for its practical success, however.

In hydrophilics, two other strategies are showing promise for increasing oxygen performance: an *increase in water content* and/or the *thinning of a lens* to increase its permeability, as shown in Figure 4 for the HEMA material discussed here.[7] Either of these strategies, however, represents a significant *benefit* (i.e., an improved corneal condition) to *risk* (optical instability and fragileness) gamble—one that only the materials chemist ultimately may be able to manage.

References

1. Terry, J.E., Hill, R.M., Human tear osmotic pressure. *Arch. Ophthal.*, 96:120, 1978.
2. Carney, L.G., Hill, R.M., Human tear pH. *Arch. Ophthal.*, 94:821, 1976.
3. Fatt, I., Freeman, R.D., Lind, D., Oxygen tension distributions in the cornea: A re-examination. *Exp. Eye Res.*, 18:357, 1974.
4. Roscoe, W.R., Hill, R.M., Corneal oxygen demand: Open eye versus closed eye conditions. *J. Fr. Ophthal.*, 1(8/9):513, 1978.
5. Polse, K.A., Mandell, R.B., Critical oxygen tension at the corneal surface. *Arch. Ophthal.*, 84:505, 1970.
6. Mandell, R.B., Fatt, I., Thinning of the cornea on awakening. *Nature*, 208:292, 1965.
7. Hill, R.M., Hydrophilic lens design: The thick and thin of it. *Excerpta Medica*, Proceedings of the Second National Symposium on Soft Contact Lenses, Chicago, August 16 and 17, 1975.

Chapter Sixteen

Behind the Closed Lid

Paradoxically, while the contact lens fitter's observations are restricted primarily to the open eye, the closed eye condition may in fact present the greatest challenges to a successful wearing outcome.

But what is known of the closed eye and the unique balances it represents? The answers to such questions are becoming increasingly important with the rapid development of *extended*-wear contact lens systems.

Expectations

Although few types of measurements have been possible so far, the very structure of the closed eye condition suggests what might be found. For example, the palpebral conjunctiva, with its warm capillary circulation, now contacts the cornea instead of the cooler atmosphere, producing temperature increases as shown in Figure 1.[1] The effect of such shifts, however, is to increase the metabolic activity of cells and, with that, their demand for oxygen.

But in place of the oxygen-laden atmosphere, the cornea must now also depend upon a much reduced level carried in those conjunctival capillaries, estimated, as shown in Figure 2, to be about one-third that of the air.[2]

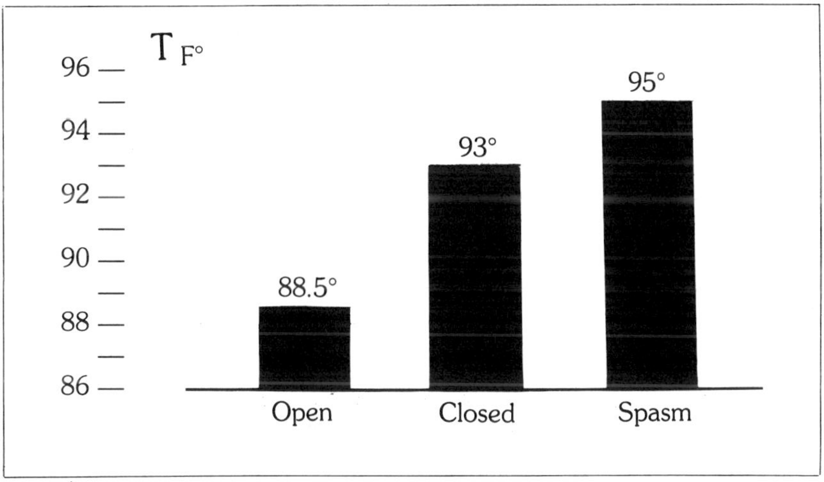

FIGURE 1. Corneal temperature when the lids are open, closed, and in blepharospasm.

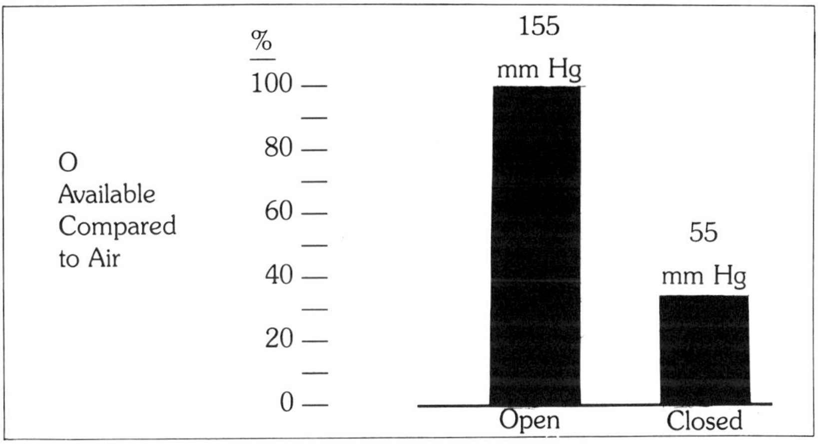

FIGURE 2. Estimated oxygen levels available to the cornea under open and closed eye conditions.

The Emerging View

In fact, measurements of oxygen demand made just after prolonged lid closure have confirmed a considerable increase in this "thirst,"[3] but such increases are generally quick to subside once the cornea has been well exposed to the atmosphere.[4]

Similarly, a more acidic tear pH has now been confirmed for the prolonged closed eye.[5] This is the result of a much reduced tear flow with the consequent buildup of metabolic byproducts and carbon dioxide,

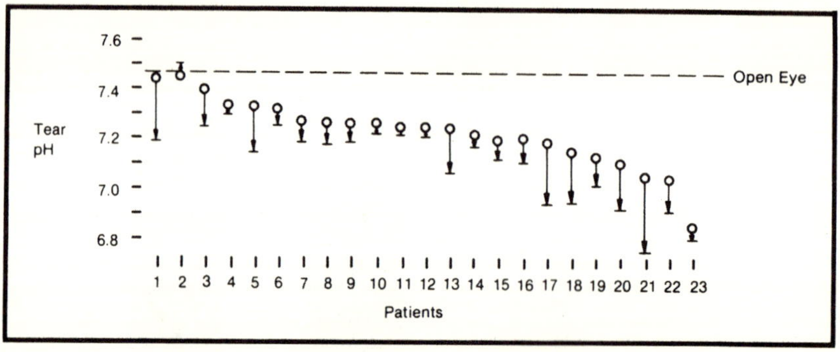

FIGURE 3. Effect of prolonged lid closure (a night of sleep) on the tear pHs of 23 patients. Their average open eye level is indicated by a dashed line; their extreme closed eye levels are indicated by the arrowheads (being more acid in almost every case).

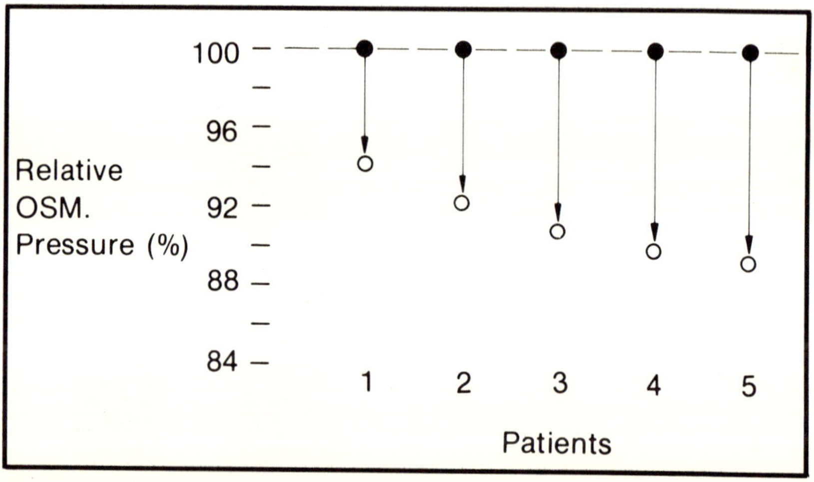

FIGURE 4. The osmotic (salt/water) balance of the tears of five patients. Their average open eye level (0.97 percent equiv. NaCl sol.) was relativized to 100 percent in each case, and the percent decrease in tear osmotic pressure under closed eye conditions is shown at the left. The average closed eye salt level was equivalent to a 0.89 percent NaCl solution.

although the degree of acid shift can vary considerably from patient to patient, as shown in Figure 3.

Finally, the reduced evaporation from a closed eye might be expected to cause a more diluted tear. This, too, has now been verified, as shown in Figure 4, although the degree of hypotonicity (i.e., dilution of salts and other solids in this extra watery tear) again varies considerably among patients, even in this pilot sample.[6] Such dilution may, of course, be the basis for corneal thickening which can be detected at awakening.[7]

The Prospects

It appears, then, that prolonged lid closure, with its several less favorable balances for the cornea, may prove to be the most challenging condition to the continuous contact lens wearer. Lenses of high oxygen permeability and low metabolic byproduct retention, however, would seem a highly promising direction to explore in pursuit of increasingly safe and acceptable *extended*-wear systems.

References

1. Hill, R.M. and A.J. Leighton, Temperature changes of human cornea and tears under a contact lens: Part I. *Am. J. Optom.*, 42:9, 1965.
2. Fatt, I. and R.D. Freeman, Oxygen tension distributions in the cornea: A re-examination. *Exp. Eye Res.*, 18:357, 1974.
3. Hill, R.M. and I. Fatt, Oxygen deprivation of the cornea by contact lenses and lid closure. *Am. J. Optom.*, 41:678, 1964.
4. Hill, R.M., Oxygen uptake of the cornea following contact lens removal. *J. Am. Optom. Assn.*, 36:913, 1965.
5. Hill, R.M. and L.G. Carney, The closed eye environment. *Am. J. Optom.*, 53:718, 1976.
6. Terry, J.E. and R.M. Hill, The osmotic variable, *J. Am. Optom. Assn.* 48:311, 1977.
7. Mandell, R.B. and I. Fatt, Thinning of the human cornea on awakening. *Nature*, 208:292, 1965.

Chapter Seventeen

How the Cornea "Takes the Heat"

Temperature may be the most variable characteristic of the cornea's environment. What impact can temperature changes have on the cornea—most especially when a contact lens is in place?

The Narrowing Aperture

Of the two covering structures, the lid and the lens, which has the greater effect on the surface temperature of the cornea?

When the surface temperature of the cornea was measured using a thermistor (a tiny, heat-sensitive electrical element),[1,2] both with and without a PMMA contact lens in place, an average temperature difference of only about 1° F was found between the two for eight human eyes studied. This rather small difference measured between the nonwearing and wearing conditions may exist because once a lens reaches corneal temperature, some tear evaporation might be expected from its front surface, as occurs with the cornea naturally.[3] Also, since a contact lens is very thin and the gradient of temperature between eye and environment is so great, some loss of heat by convection and radiation should be taking place, too.

In contrast, however, when the lid was closed over a contact lens, the temperature often rose several degrees. Figure 1 shows this rise in tear-corneal temperature as the lid aperture was reduced in measured

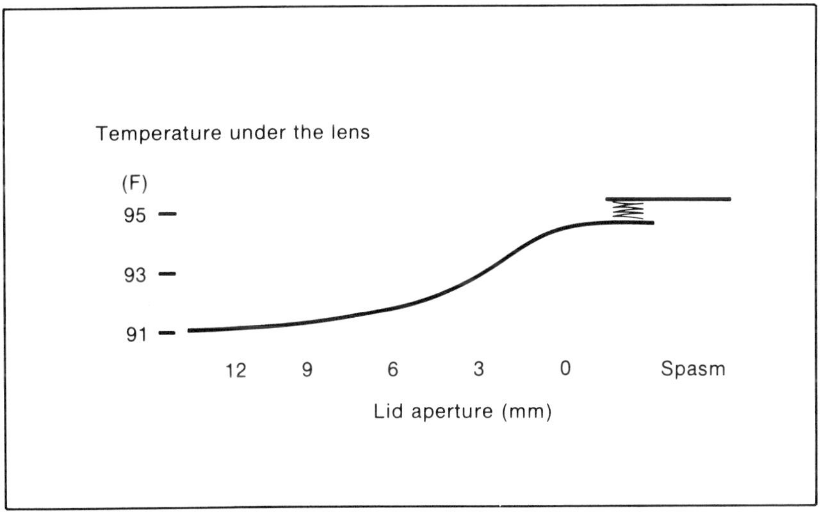

FIGURE 1. The increase in tear-cornea temperature under a contact lens as the lid is gradually closed and during blepharospasm.

steps. Highest temperatures were recorded during blepharospasms, when atmospheric shielding of the cornea and lens by the lid was combined with circulatory warmth of the palpebral conjunctival surface now in direct contact with the eye-lens system, plus the presence of added lid "muscle heat" due to the intense spasmic activity.

Response to Temperature Increase

But are there likely to be clinical consequences from temperature increases such as those shown in Figure 1? At least potentially, *yes.* The most significant response the mammalian cornea makes to a rise in temperature is to speed up its metabolism,[4,5] hence its demand for oxygen under the contact lens. With relaxed lid closure, an increase of 10 to 15 percent might be expected, and even more during periods of blepharospasm (Figure 2).

The Price of Overtaxation

What, then, are the clinical circumstances where an increased temperature and oxygen demand might overtax a marginally performing lens-tear pump?

Two examples are the poorly adapted patient who is prone to noticeable lid squint while wearing his lenses and the patient who persists in reading for extended periods with no regular relief. In both cases, the narrowed lid aperture and increased temperature and oxygen demand

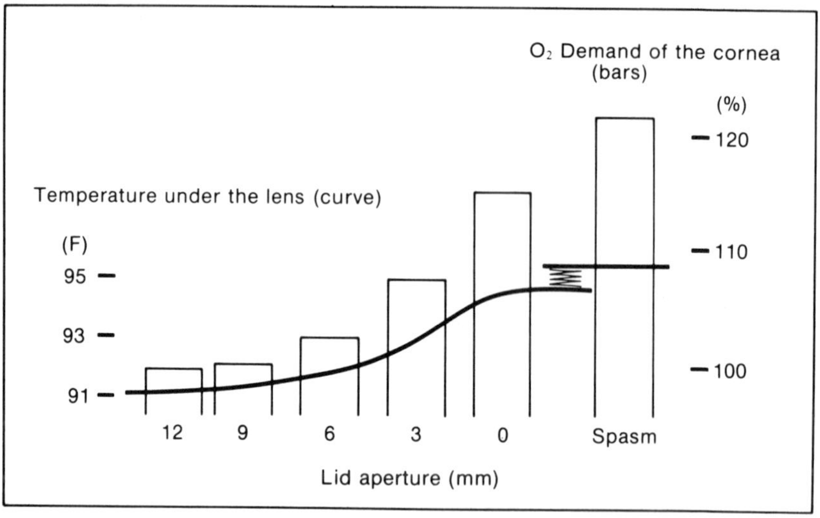

FIGURE 2. The commensurate increase in oxygen demand by the cornea as the temperature under a contact lens increases.

may be enough to cause a chronic irritation, threshold edema, and a generally compromised visual performance.

Very possibly, the temperature effects of prolonged lid closure associated with sleep may prove to be one of the ultimate challenges of the extended contact lens wear regimes.

References

1. Hill, R.M., Leighton, A.J., Temperature changes of human cornea and tears under a contact lens: I. *Amer. J. Optom*, 42:9-16, 1965.
2. Hill, R.M., Leighton, A.J., Temperature changes of human cornea and tears under a contact lens: II. *Amer. J. Optom.*, 42:72-77, 1965.
3. Moses, R.A., Ed., *Adler's Physiology of the Eye*, ed. 6. St. Louis: C.V. Mosby Company, 1975, pp. 21, 50.
4. Hill, R.M., Schoessler, J.P., Fatt, I., Oxygen flux across the environmental interface of teleost cornea. *Nature*, 214:384-385, 1967.
5. Freeman, R.D., Fatt, I., Environmental influences on ocular temperature. *Invest. Ophthal.*, 12:596-602, 1973.

Chapter Eighteen

Oxygen Demand: The Same for Every Cornea?

When faced with persistent edema, it is not uncommon for a fitter to wonder: Could this cornea be making "unreasonable" (unusually high) demands for oxygen?

Do, indeed, some corneas have greater demands than others? Because corneas may be of different thicknesses (i.e., composed of different numbers of epithelial layers and cell totals), different ages (i.e., with different rates of mitotic activity), and different histories (in terms of health and trauma), such a concept may not be unrealistic. Are the tolerances for relative starvation (e.g., under a nonoxygen or low-oxygen permeable contact lens) the same for every cornea? To what degree might the oxygen demands of a patient's cornea dictate clinical success or failure?

Three Profiles

To explore these questions, three patients with diverse (conventional PMMA) contact lens backgrounds were studied.[1] The first had no regular wearing history (due to a low refractive error) but was known from previous research studies to be a very tolerant wearer. The second was a newly adapted wearer, with a full-time wearing history of about one month. The third was a model contact lens wearer of some eight years. All were in their 20's at the time of the study.

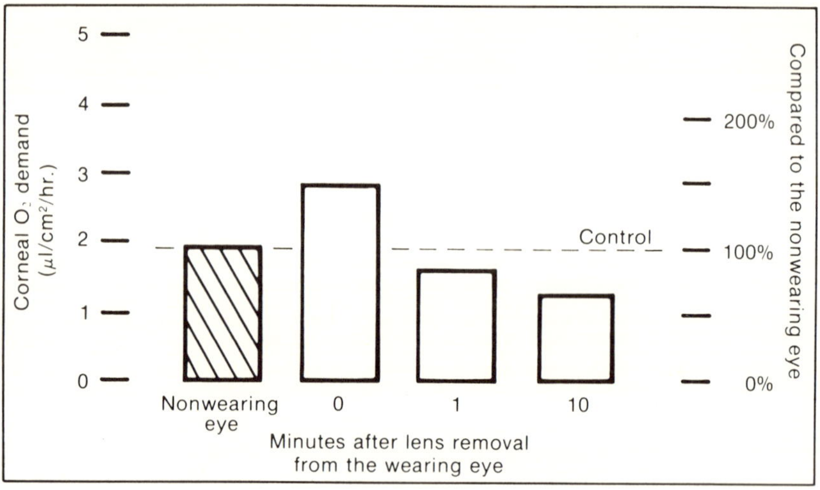

FIGURE 1. A nonadapted patient. The oxygen demand of this patient's nonwearing cornea (shaded bar) compared to his wearing cornea (for an eight-hour period) immediately following lens removal (i.e., at zero minutes) and at one and 10 minutes later. (Polyethylene probe reservoir)

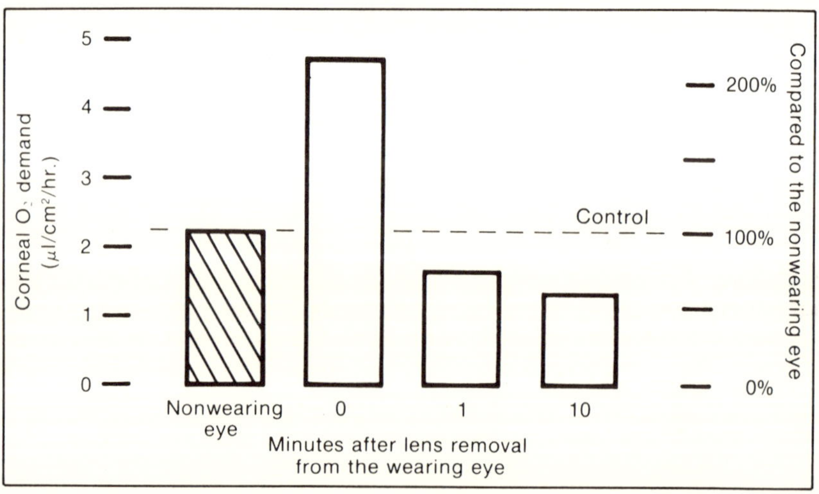

FIGURE 2. A recently adapted successful wearer. The oxygen demand of this patient's nonwearing cornea (shaded bar) compared to his wearing cornea (for an eight-hour period) immediately following lens removal (i.e., at zero minutes) and at one minute and 10 minutes later. (Polyethylene probe reservoir)

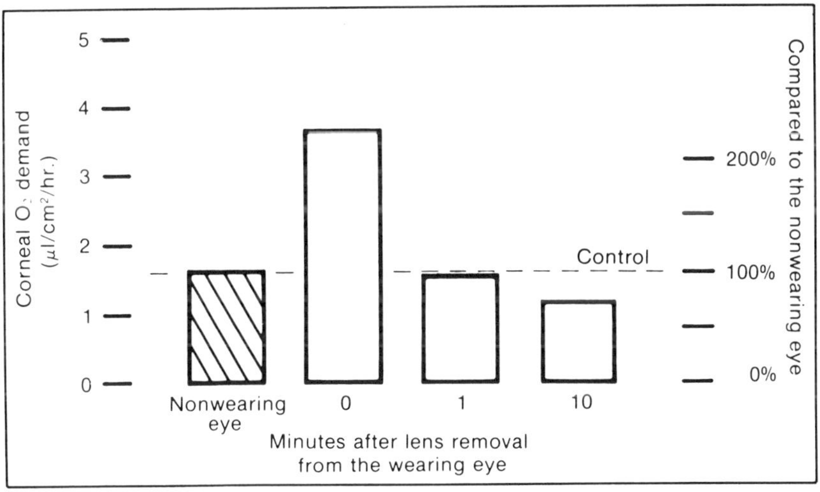

FIGURE 3. A very successful eight-year veteran wearer. The oxygen demand of this patient's nonwearing cornea (shaded bar) compared to his wearing cornea (for an eight-hour period) immediately following lens removal (i.e., at zero minutes) and at one minute and 10 minutes later. (Polyethylene probe reservoir)

During the eight-hour period before these measurements, there was no lens on one eye, while a K fitted (within 0.50D of the flattest meridian) lens was worn on the other eye. No cornea in the group had more than 0.50D of astigmatism. The methods and reservoir calculation models used have been described earlier.[2,3]

Immediately following that period of normal waking hour activity, i.e., at zero minutes, the oxygen demands of both eyes were measured at their central corneal points. The responses of the eyes wearing lenses were measured at one minute and at 10 minutes following lens removal. Figures 1 through 3 summarize those findings for the three patients studied, while Figure 4 represents the "composite wearer," based on the averaged findings of the three.

The Tortoises and the Hare

Among those features common to every case were the following:

(1) Each cornea from which a lens had been removed showed a marked increase in its demand for oxygen compared to that of its nonwearing mate. This is seemingly indicative of a sustained relative anoxia maintained under those lenses *in situ*.

(2) By one minute following lens removal, however, the oxygen demand of each had returned to the level of its nonwearing mate, and by 10 minutes following removal, their demands were significantly below that

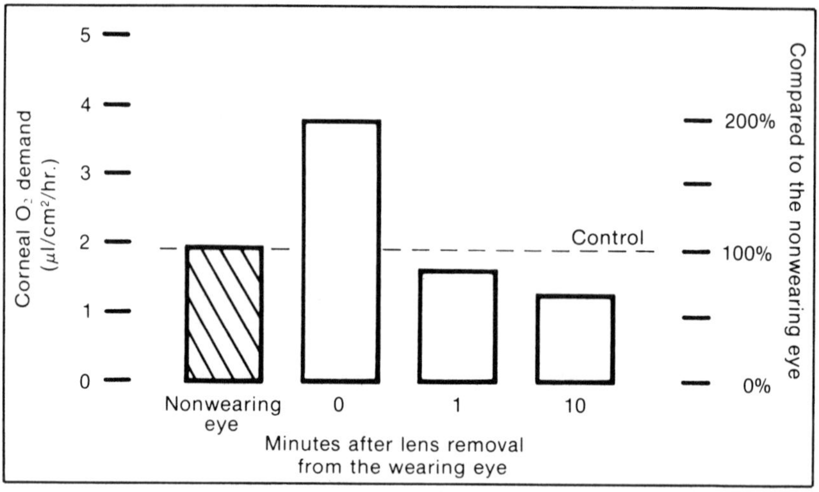

FIGURE 4. A "composite wearer" (based on the averages for the group). The oxygen demand of the nonwearing cornea (shaded bar) compared to the wearing cornea (for an eight-hour period) immediately following lens removal (i.e., at zero minutes) and at one minute and 10 minutes later. (Polyethylene probe reservoir)

level (a kind of "reactive depression"). The initial increase in oxygen demand is due in part to the refilling of adjacent oxygen depleted tissues previously drained by the epithelium (e.g., the stroma). The later period of "reactive depression" may be due to the presence of an anoxia-based edema (i.e., due to the additional epithelial water through which basal and other internally contained cells must "pull" their oxygen).

However, could success in fitting still be based to some degree on a talent for sorting the tortoises from the hares? Although not yet fully answered, dependence on such a differentiation should, in any event, progressively lessen as more efficient oxygen permeable lenses continue to appear.

Note—Polyethylene probe reservoirs commonly give absolute oxygen uptake values for the cornea equal to one half or less those found for saline probe reservoirs (possibly due to constants' inaccuracies, in need of refinement for polyethylene).

References

1. Hill, R.M., Oxygen uptake of the cornea following contact lens removal. *J. Amer. Optom. Assoc.*, 36(10):913, 1965.
2. Hill, R.M., Fatt, I., Oxygen depletion of a limited reservoir by human. *Nature*, 200:1011, 1963.
3. Hill, R.M., Fatt, I., Oxygen uptake from a reservoir of limited volume by the human cornea *in vivo*. *Science*, 142:1295, 1963.

Chapter Nineteen

Conjunctival Competition?

Certainly the cornea's role as an oxygen consumer is well appreciated by the contact lens practitioner, but is this the only tissue in the contact lens system with such needs?

Supply and Demand

It is not likely! In fact, the conjunctiva has a considerably greater surface area than the cornea and also is covered with oxygen-demanding epithelial cells. This was reported over 15 years ago in a study in which the oxygen uptake of the bulbar conjunctiva was compared with that of an inert surface (leather), skin on the forearm and the cornea. Those observations, summarized in Figure 1, contain at least two points of special interest: (1) human bulbar conjunctiva can have an oxygen uptake rate that may rival the cornea and (2) the rate of oxygen uptake by a particular patch of conjunctiva can depend on its location (e.g., how near it is to the limbus).

One reason for this latter variation could be the particular density and proximity of conjunctival blood vessels to the spot being measured. Since the oxygen tension in conjunctival capillaries is only one-third (or less) that in air, those capillaries, when presented with an oxygen-laden (air) reservoir, may draw vigorously from it, at least until that source is exhausted down to that level the capillaries themselves contain. The

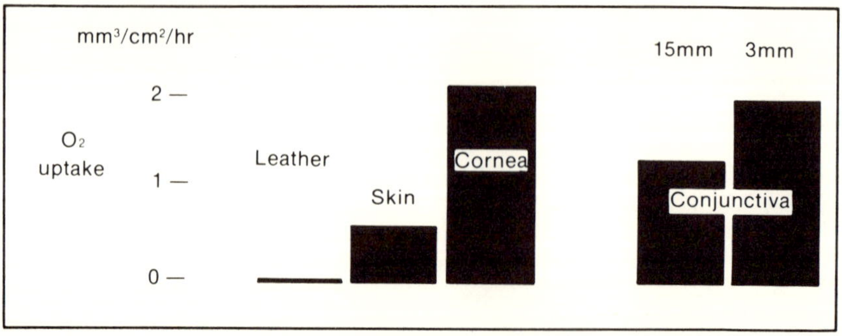

FIGURE 1. Relative oxygen demands of human conjunctiva (3mm and 15mm from the limbus) as compared to an inert surface (leather), skin of the forearm, and human cornea. (Polyethylene probe reservoir)

closer the vessels to the site measured or the greater their number, the more substantial an attractor of oxygen they would represent.

Source or Sink?

These observations suggest then, as Figure 2 shows schematically, that depending on the amount of oxygen reaching the tears, the conjunctiva might act as a *source* of oxygen for the cornea (as in the closed lid case wherein the tear level is very low) or as a *sink* for oxygen (as in the open eye condition, where high levels directly from the atmosphere prevail).

A "Slice Off the Top"?

An interesting clinical question then might be: When in its role as a sink might the conjunctiva become a significant competitor to the cornea for available oxygen carried in the tears?

The answer ultimately depends on what the practitioner believes the minimum adequate amount of oxygen for the cornea to be. If for some reason the level chosen were 10 percent oxygen (versus 21 percent in air), then the conjunctiva, which itself has a capillary level of only 3 to 7 percent, would be at the low (i.e., consuming) end of the gradient and must be considered a competitor for oxygen under the "rarefied" conditions of, for example, an impermeable scleral contact lens.

However, if the edema detection level of Polse and Mandell (approximately 2 percent oxygen) is taken as a possible minimum, the conjunctiva at 3 to 7 percent would be at the upper (i.e., contributing) end of the gradient and would have to be considered a benefactor to the cornea's needs.

Until more is known of the specifics of corneal oxygen requirement (on both short and very long-term bases), the precise answer to this

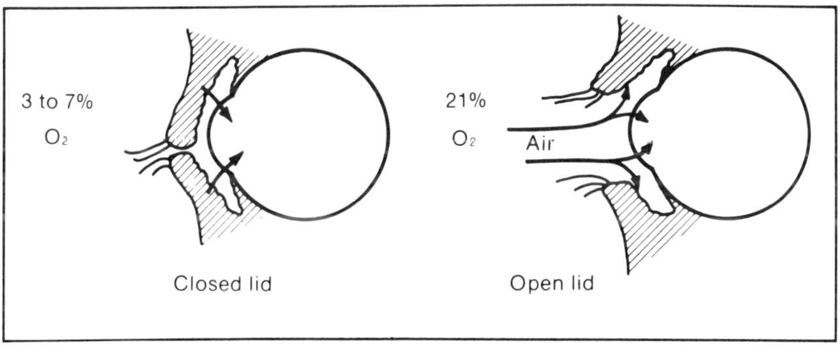

FIGURE 2. The conjunctiva as an oxygen source for the cornea during closed lid conditions, and as an oxygen sink or competitor with the cornea under open lid conditions.

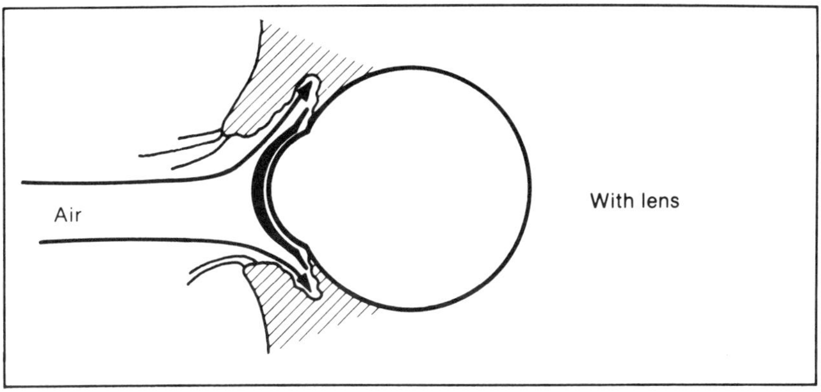

FIGURE 3. The conjunctiva as a potential competitor to the cornea for oxygen entering a contact lens system.

question of conjunctival competition remains philosophical. There would seem to be at least some consolation to the fitter in the interim, however. Most modern materials and designs do function tolerably well in the presence of this seldom-mentioned tissue partner, suggesting that preliminary design negotiations with it have been generally successful.

Note—Polyethylene probe reservoirs give oxygen uptake values for the cornea which are about one half or less than those found with saline reservoirs (possibly due to constants' inaccuracies, in need of refinement for polyethylene).

References

1. Hill, R.M., Fatt, I., Oxygen depletion of a limited reservoir by human conjunctiva. *Nature* 200:1011, 1963.
2. Fatt, I., Freeman, R.D., Lin. D., Oxygen tension distributions in the cornea: A reexamination *Exp. Eye. Res.*, 18:357, 1974.
3. Polse, K.A., Mandell, R.B., Critical oxygen tension at the corneal surface. *Arch. Ophthal.*, 84:505, 1970.

Chapter Twenty

For the Connoisseurs of Blink

After all that has been said and written about the blink, could there be any mysteries remaining?

Alas, yes . . . perhaps the most fundamental question of them all remains: what is the blink's quantitative worth in a contact lens system? It is at this point that even the most sophisticated of fitters seems to grow reluctant when pressed for a number: 50 percent, 20 percent, 70 percent, . . . 5 percent, as a tear exchange volume per blink?

The "Sodium Scheme"

Although clinically this volume exchange problem remains a technically resistant one, there is at least one laboratory method that can give us a fair approximation of the answer on an individual lens-eye basis. It is an approach designed by Cuklanz and Hill in 1969,[1] whose strategy is reviewed schematically in Figure 1, A through D. It requires at the outset the filling of the lens bowl with a high concentration of some nonconsumable but naturally occurring particles in tears such as sodium.

Suppose then, as in part A of our schema, that 100 sodium particles (ions) were trapped under the lens at the time of insertion and that a similar volume of tears in the outside tear pool would contain only 10 particles. Let us suppose, too, that a blink causes a 10 percent tear exchange with this lens design. If one can then imagine an equal pair of

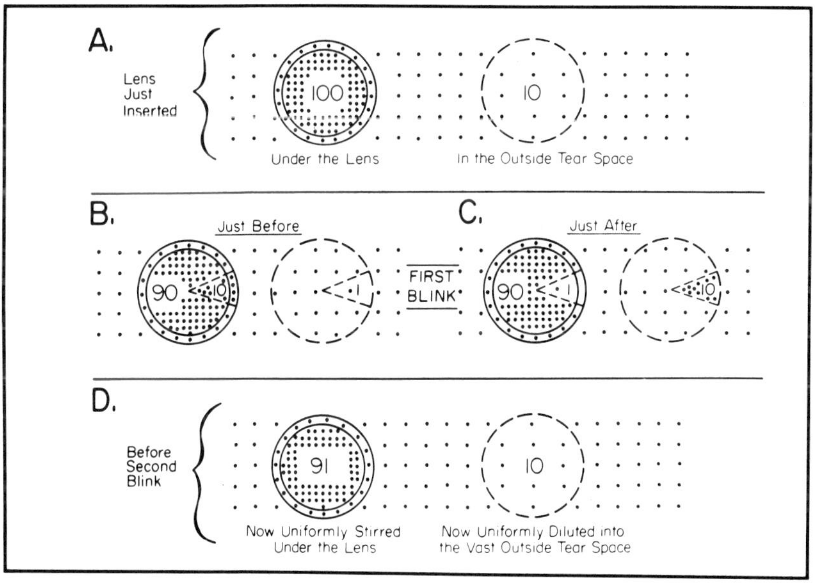

FIGURE 1. A schematic representation of the phases and volumes of tear exchange between the contact lens and outside tear pools (see text).

such volumes, as in part B, with one under the lens containing 10 sodium particles and the other in the outside tear space containing one sodium particle, then the first blink should bring about an exchange as shown in part C. Finally during the interblink period (i.e., before the second blink takes place), as shown in part D, the particles now remaining under the lens, 91, should be uniformly redistributed, as will those discharged into the outside tear pool. That outside pool is so vast, however, that the concentration of those sodium particles discharged from under the lens is quickly dissipated down to the original outside tear pool level, shown as 10 in our illustration.

For Those Who Prefer Equations

If we label each of the particle pools in Figure 1, they can then be assembled into the following equation:

$$N_I = (1 - e)\, N_0 + eN_T \qquad (1)$$

in which N_0 equals the number of particles under the lens before the first blink occurs (equals 100 here, as in A of Figure 1); N_T equals the number of particles in a similar volume of tears outside the lens (equals 10 here, also as in A of Figure 1); e equals pump exchange factor (taken as 0.1, or 10 percent of the tear volume under the lens, as in B and C of

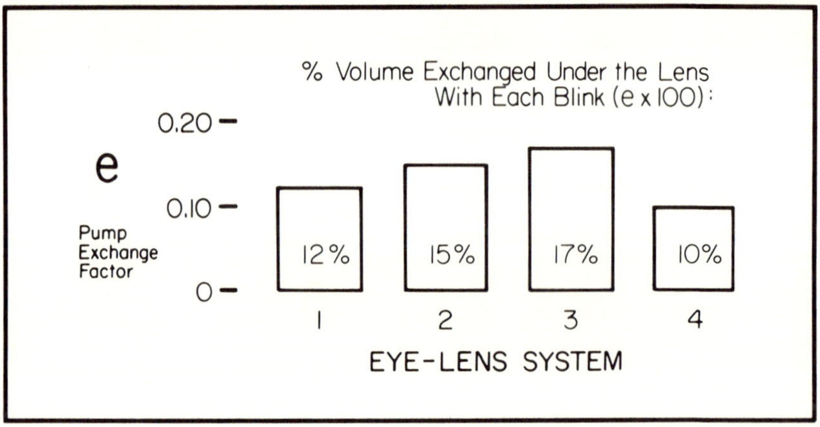

FIGURE 2. The e values and percentages of tear volumes exchanged under the lens with each blink (e × 100), calculated for four human eye-contact lens systems based on measurements of sodium ions in their tears (see text).

Figure 1); and N_I equals the net number of particles remaining under the lens following blink 1 (predicted to equal 91 here, as in D of Figure 1). Solving this equation for N_I then:

$$N_I = (1 - 0.1)\ 100 + 0.1\ (10) = 91 \qquad (2)$$

which is the number predicted to be left after that first blink.*

Of primary interest to us here, however, is to rearrange this equation so that, given N_O, N_T, and N_I we could determine what e, the pump exchange factor for a particular lens-eye system, would be. By algebraically moving the terms of Equation 1 around, the result then is as follows:

$$e = (N_O - N_I)/(N_O - N_T) \qquad (3)$$

Inserting the values from Figure 1 into this relationship gives the following:

$$e = (100 - 91)/(100 - 10) = 9/90 = 0.1 \qquad (4)$$

If e is then multiplied by 100, the percentage of the lens tear pool exchanged per blink is obtained, equal here to 10 percent.

---

*The equation for more than one blink expands as follows:

$$N_n = (1 - e)^n N_O + eN_T\ [(1 - e)^{n-1} + (1 - e)^{n-2} + \ldots + 1]$$

These equations do not allow for backflow of some part of the stagnant tears in under the lens again and thus represent a first approximation that will be in error by that amount.

TABLE 1
Physical characteristics of the four lens systems.

System	Corneal radius (mm)	Lens base curve (mm)	Lens diameter (mm)
1	7.77 × 7.70	7.70	9.70
2	7.78 × 7.75	7.75	9.70
3	8.02 × 7.83	7.80	9.70
4	8.02 × 7.83	7.80	9.70

Putting Theory into Practice

With the strategies above and being able to measure N_0, N_T, and N_I in the case of sodium by a quantitative method of flame photometry, the e values for four lens-eye systems were calculated. Figure 2 shows the distribution of e values found among them (see also Table 1).

It appears then for the particular type of contact lens system studied here that exchange values of from 10 to 17 percent per blink were represented, although allowing for backflow effects even these efficiencies would be rated just a bit high. In fact follow-up oxygen measurements made on these corneas did reveal an increased demand for oxygen on lens removal over their normal nonwearing levels.

Although these corneas may be able to physiologically tolerate such exchange levels at normal blink frequencies, clearly the ideal e values, i.e., those that would produce no increased oxygen demand, are somewhat higher and for now must still be gauged by those most practical clinical criteria: relief of all of the patient's detectable signs and symptoms.

Reference

1. Cuklanz, M.D., Hill, R.M., Oxygen requirements of the contact lens system. *Amer. J. Optom.*, 46:228, 1969.

Chapter Twenty-One

Epithelial Injury

Of the many possibilities that may interrupt contact lens wear, surely epithelial injury commands the most respect. Together with being the most powerful and therefore the most optically vital interface to the eye, the corneal epithelium is, of course, the most vulnerable.

However, it is the immediate management problem of epithalial injury that presents the greatest challenge to the contact lens fitter. For example, how soon is it safe to return a lens to such an eye? Most particularly, how adequate is the clearance of slit-lamp signs as a clinical gauge of recovery?

Into the Pits

Although not yet available in practice, one of the most revealing measures of epithelial normalcy in the laboratory is the amount of oxygen that a tissue demands.[1] While the normal corneal surface is not completely uniform in this regard, the vast central expanse of it takes in amounts deviating as little as 5 percent from its overall mean, as shown in Figure 1. The very center is the greatest exception, at 6.5 percent less than the overall mean, but since it is also the coolest part of the corneal surface, its demand should be lowest as well. (The cooler a cell is, the slower is its metabolism and the less will be its demand for oxygen.[2])

Suppose, however, that we explore the worst case of epithelial loss

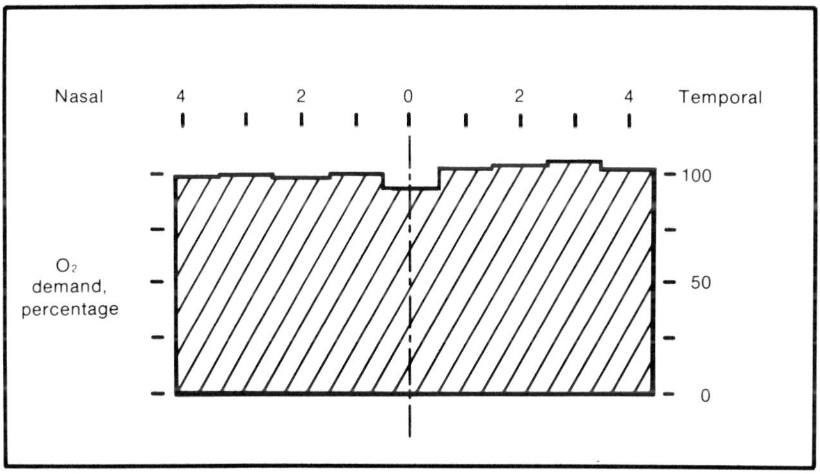

FIGURE 1. Oxygen demands at several sites across a representative diameter of a normal cornea.

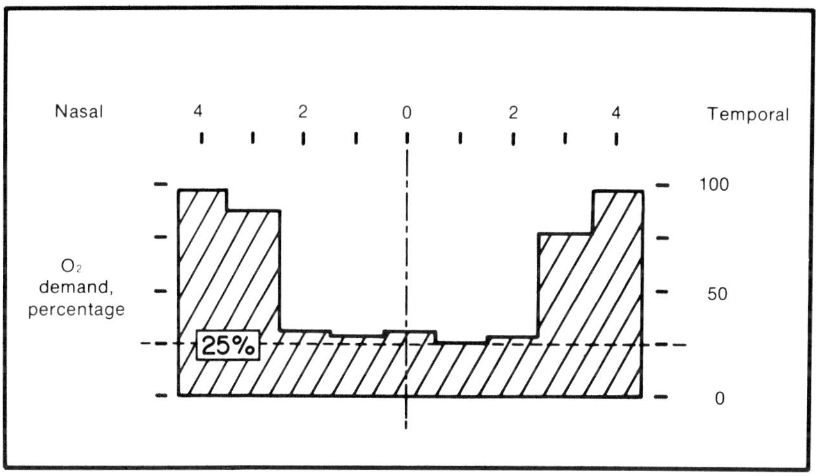

FIGURE 2. The immediate sharp decrease in oxygen demand within a region of central cornea just denuded of epithelium all the way down to the stroma.

(i.e., all the way down to the stroma) and follow how such a lesion—say 5mm in diameter—and its annual surround recover. A fall in oxygen uptake across a representative diameter of this wound and its surround is shown in Figure 2. Most surprising, perhaps, is that the demand for oxygen does not fall completely to zero across the lesion floor. This

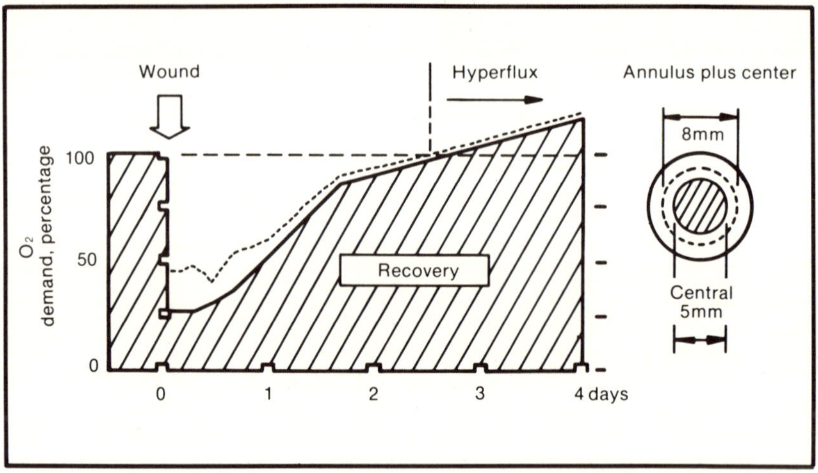

FIGURE 3. The fall and subsequent recovery of oxygen demand of the center (shaded) and surrounding annulus plus the center (dotted) areas of the wound back to the prewound level within three days. A hyperflux (extra demand) developed beyond (see text). The area between the solid and the dotted curves represents the net oxygen demand of the annulus itself, whose activity is closest and most vital to the healing of the central lesion.

remaining inflow (some 25 percent of the normal) is most likely due to both stromal cell consumption and an inward leakage down the steep gradient between the high oxygen level in the atmosphere and the much lower level present in the aqueous humor.

Physiological Ghosts

How long will recovery take? Figure 3 shows the persistent climb back to the normal level (labeled 100) for the 5mm-diameter lesion area; nearly three days (72 hours) are required, however. The immediate surround (1.5mm-wide annulus) also shows some initial effects but recovers in two and one-half to three days as well. Both zones then persist in showing a hyperflux (greater than original demand) for an extended period (monitored up to 122 hours) beyond.

Of particular clinical interest here is that all slit-lamp signs disappeared well before the 122-hour point, when the residual hyperflux still prevailed. One can at present only guess at the cause of this extra oxygen inflow. It might possibly be an aftereffect of the massive cell divison and migration required to rebuild such a wound area and to replenish normal reserves. In view of the presence of this extra oxygen inflow, however, it seems at minimum a clinically prudent strategy to give the cornea just a little extra recovery time even after slit-lamp signs have disappeared. Considering the long-term risks of tissue compromise and complications, a day or two further delay before resuming lens wear is a relatively small price for the additional safety it represents.

References

1. Hill, R.M., Keates, R.M., Quantifying epithelial healing of the cornea, *in vivo. Arch. Ophthal.*, 82:675, 1969.

2. Hill, R.M., Schoessler, J., Fatt, I., Oxygen flux across the environmental interface of teleost cornea. *Nature.*, 214:384, 1967.

Chapter Twenty-Two

Anesthetic Impact

There are occasions when an anesthetic must be placed in the eye, particularly with the older contact lens patient during Goldmann tonometry, gonioscopy, or the Schirmer II tear test, to cite just a few examples. How soon after such a disturbance is normal corneal function restored? Do such recoveries differ markedly among anesthetics? Based on signs of metabolic activity, how soon can a contact lens be returned to the eye?

Physiological Downtime

Augsburger[1] made parallel measurements of both corneal sensation and oxygen uptake—the latter being one of the more sensitive physiological indicators of anoxia, edema, and trauma.[2,3,4]

Cocaine, which in 1884 was the first anesthetic applied directly to the cornea, has earned the most infamous reputation for aftereffects. Consequently, this substance provides us the most vivid profile of physiological disturbance.[5,6] As indicated in Figure 1, at the dosage level required to achieve 30 minutes of maximum analgesia (4 drops of a 1 percent solution*), the impact on epithelial cell activity is considerable, as

*The average drop volume for the applicator was the following: cocaine, 48mm^3; tetracaine, 48mm^3; and benoxinate, 25mm^3. A mm^3 volume is also called a microliter (μl) or a lambda.

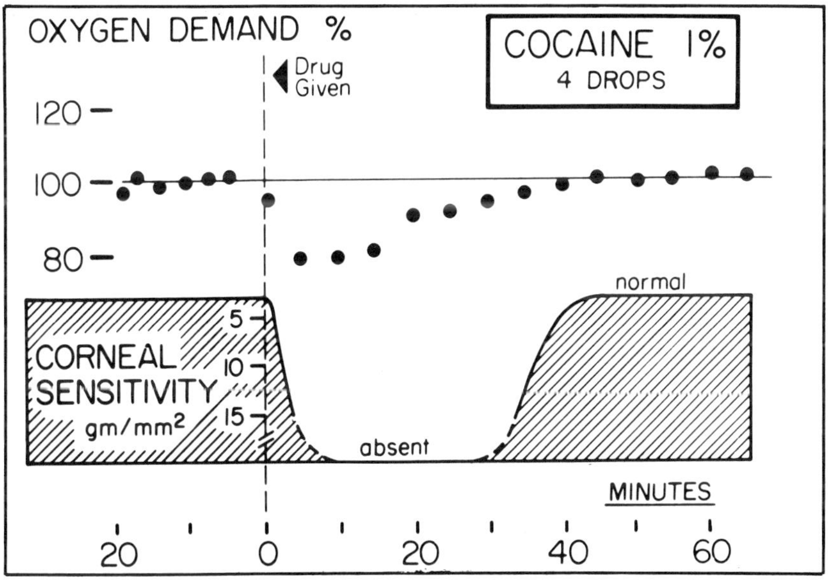

FIGURE 1. The time periods of corneal insensitivity and reduced oxygen uptake resulting from a 4-drop dose of 1 percent cocaine.

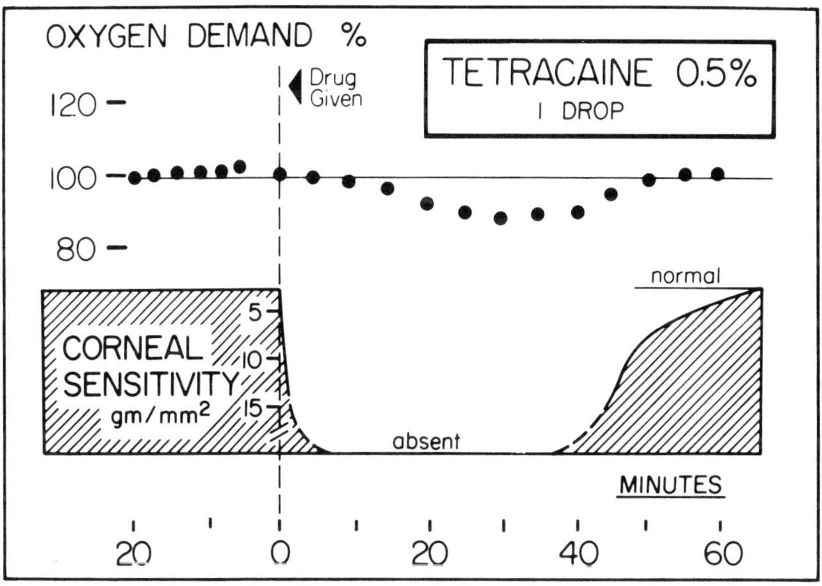

FIGURE 2. The time periods of corneal insensitivity and reduced oxygen uptake resulting from a 1-drop dose of 0.5 percent tetracaine.

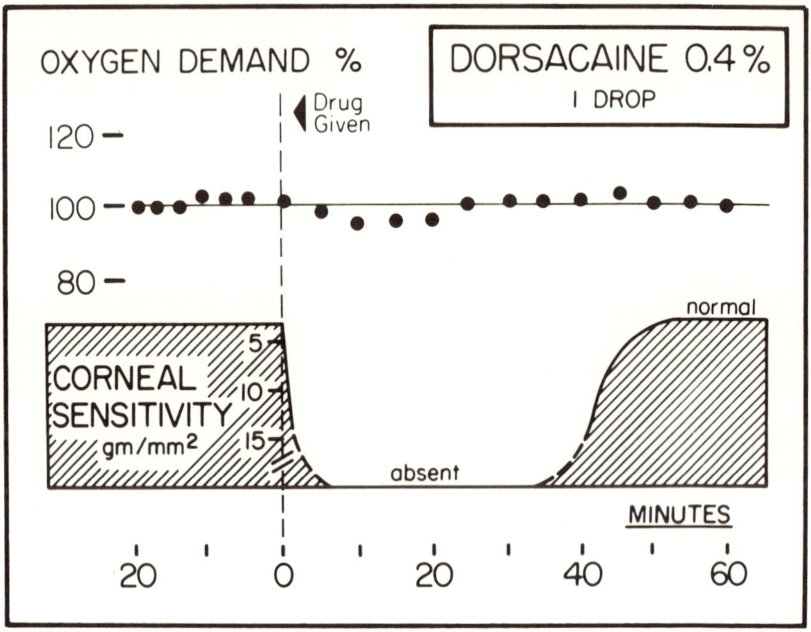

FIGURE 3. The time periods of corneal insensitivity and reduced oxygen uptake resulting from a 1-drop dose of 0.4 percent Dorsacaine (benoxinate hydrochloride).

shown by a 20 percent decline in oxygen uptake.

In contrast, tetracaine, the drug now used more frequently, can achieve a similar analgesic interval with only a single drop of 0.5 percent concentration (Figure 2). Even more important from a physiological point of view is the less severe effect this agent appears to have on oxygen-dependent mechanisms of the cornea.

Most clinically effective is the corneal anesthetic Dorsacaine (benoxinate hydrochloride). While only 1 drop of 0.4 percent concentration results in a very similar analgesic span to tetracaine, Dorsacaine's impact on aerobic (oxygen-dependent) metabolism is considerably less and passes even more quickly, as shown in Figure 3. Also, as Polse, Keener, and Jauregui point out, even lower dosage levels may be fully adequate for such procedures as tonometry.[7]

Other Influences to Consider

The fitter must also take into account the supplementary components in packaged units, which can add their own (although somewhat lesser) contributions to the physiological disturbances described. Benzalkonium chloride, an often-included germicide, can itself influence corneal penetration rates.[8] Different combinations of various germicides, buffering agents, and other additives acting together with the primary analgesic agent may shift the Augsburger curves (Figures 1 through 3) accordingly.

Clinical Overview

Considerable progress has been made in the development of modern anesthetic drugs that can achieve reasonable periods of sustained analgesia with significantly less depression of oxygen-related corneal processes. Nevertheless, a minimum of perhaps twice the time required for the full return of sensation is appropriate before lens reinsertion to compensate for patient variations and to gain a fuller assurance of the cornea's capacity to cope once again with the wearing environment.

References

1. Augsburger, A.R., and Hill, R.M., Corneal anesthetics and epithelial oxygen flux, *Arch. Ophthal.*, 88:305, 1972.
2. Hill, R.M., and Fatt, I., Oxygen requirements under a contact lens, *American J. of Optom.*, 41:382, 1964.
3. Hill, R.M., and Schoessler, J.P., Epithelial edema: Respiratory characteristics of the Lesion, *Amer. J. of Optom.*, 45:241, 1968.
4. Hill, R.M., and Keates, R.H., Quantifying epithelial healing of the cornea *in vivo.*, *Arch. Ophthal.*, 82:675, 1969.
5. Duke-Elder, S., *System of Ophthalmology*. Vol. VII: The Foundations of Pharmacology, C.V. Mosby Co., St. Louis, 1962, p. 595.
6. Behrendt, T., Corneal lesions after topical anesthesia, *Amer. J. Ophtal.*, 41:99, 1956.
7. Polse, K.A., Keener, R.J., and Jauregui, M.J., Dose-Response effects of corneal anesthetics, *Amer. J. of Optom. and Physio. Optics* 55:8, 1978.
8. Havener, W. I., *Ocular Pharmacology*, C.V. Mosby Co., St. Louis, 1974, p. 418.

Part III: THE LENS

The lens as a foreign body: Old and new properties; continuing vulnerabilities; and some of the subtle aspects of care and neglect.

Chapter Twenty-Three

The Hard Lens as a Foreign Body

Even the most well-designed hard lens, when inserted into the average eye, is destined to draw a response of "sustained awareness." But the sequence of events underlying that symptom and its related signs (lid margin irritation, reflex tearing, and corneal edema) have now moved well beyond the predictions of the experienced practitioner. In fact, several links in that response chain have already been successfully monitored and measured as they happen, for example, the initial irritation of the lid margin (followed by its ultimate "toughening" with wearing time)[1] as well as the pachometric tracking of corneal edema with contact lens wear.[2]

Now one further link, the bridge between the two above, has given way to quantitative scrutiny: those delicate balances of particles (ions, enzymes, nutrients, metabolites, etc.) within the tears. This feature is most vulnerable to lid margin irritation and can dicate the swelling of the cornea and its clinical compromise in health and performance.

A "Numbers Game"

Of the several causes of corneal swelling including trauma, oxygen starvation, and osmotic (particle) imbalances, the latter can play a very prominent role in the initial adaptation. Since water is attracted to high concentrations of particles, it is clinically advantageous to maintain

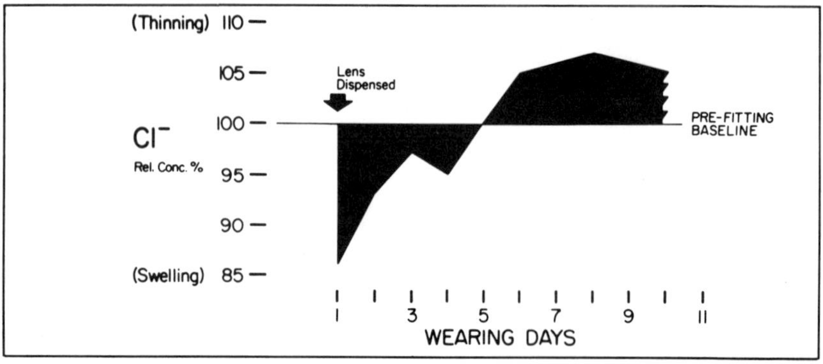

FIGURE 1. Change in tear chloride levels (shown in black) *as a patient adapts to a hard (PMMA) contact lens (modified from Schmidt et al.*[3]*).*

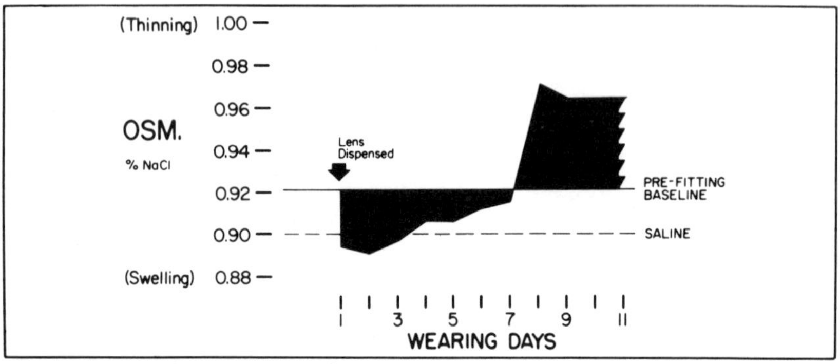

FIGURE 2. Changes in tear osmotic pressure (shown in black) *as a patient adapts to hard (PMMA) contact lenses (modified from Terry and Hill*[5]*).*

particle-rich tears (rather than to allow water to be attracted into the corneal epithelial cells).

One quickly realizes that the most valuable "players" in this game of concentration are the smallest of the tear particles, the salt ions, since greater numbers of them can be packed into a small volume of tears than any other kind—and density draws water as if in an insatiable effort to dilute its particles.

As a clinical test of this physiological expectation, we might follow the presence of the chloride ion (Figure 1). The baseline we will work from is the prefitting average of this particle in this patient's tears (called 100 percent here) as it was measured throughout the waking periods of several days prior to dispensing.[3] Notice the effect on these particles, however, when the patients' lens (conventional PMMA) was dispensed. The precipitous fall is also indicative of what is happening to many tear

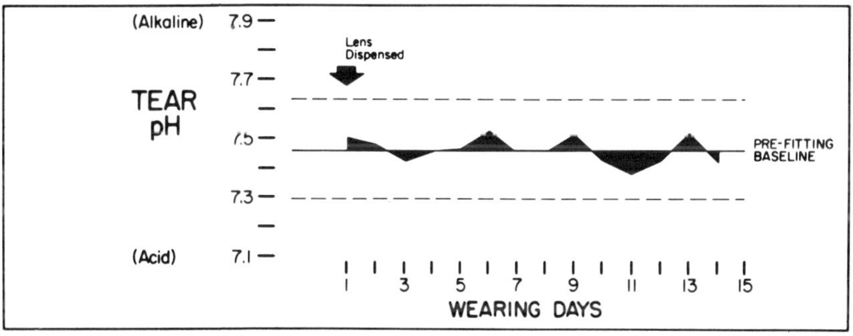

*FIGURE 3. Tear pH changes of an average patient (*shown in black*) during adaptation to hard (PMMA) contact lenses (modified from Carney and Hill*[6]*).* Broken lines *indicate the 1SD limits from the prefitting baseline.*

particles (i.e., the result of an abrupt dilution by "reflex" or defense tears of a very "watery" nature).[4]

Water in these dilute tears would then, by our "rule" of particle dilution (i.e., water will move toward more concentrated particles), be drawn very rapidly and forcibly into the cornea and result in edema and its effects of photophobia, reduced resolution, etc.

In this patient's case, however, the lids began to "toughen"; sensation was reduced, as was reflex tear flow, and by the fifth wearing day the prefitting baseline was successfully regained, with edema and its attendant symptoms resolved. In fact, the ultimate tear chloride level established for this patient was somewhat "saltier" than before fitting, a fairly common outcome.

The Effect "In Concert"

While the chloride and the other prominent ions (sodium, calcium, bicarbonate, etc.) do make the most prominent osmotic contributions to the tears, larger components (such as lipids and proteins) add their influence as well. The total effect of all contributing particles, the osmotic pressure, can also be measured as adaptation to hard lenses takes place.[4] Figure 2 illustrates that the "in-concert" behavior of those many contributing particles does, as might be predicted, follow the "chloride course" fairly closely,[5] even to the mild "overshoot" (hypertonic) end result—which, in terms of diminishing edema, is distinctly to the practitioner's advantage.

A Notable Exception?

Among the many tear components, however, there may be at least one exception that seems to show little or no significant change in the average patient's tears during hard lens adaptation: the hydrogen ion.[6] As shown in Figure 3, only minor drift occurred for the population studied from the prefitting baseline, resulting in very little net shift in tear pH. Such stability should again be to the practitioner's advantage, since a sufficient fall in pH (an acid shift) can be the basis for discomfort[7] or even cause for a depression in oxygen uptake by the cornea.[6]

Toward a Swift and Tolerable Result

The mechanisms underlying the "foreign body reaction" to a hard contact lens are giving way to objective analysis. Yet such quantitative monitoring can now only serve to further substantiate the practitioner's observations and to perhaps lend a bit of "moral" support to his prognostic and management decisions.

References

1. Lowther, G.E., Hill, R.M., Sensitivity thresholds of the lower lid margin in the course of adaptation to contact lenses. Amer. J. Optom., 45:587, 1968.
2. Harris, M.G., Mandell, R.B., Contact lens adaptation: Osmotic theory. Amer. J. Optom., 46:196, 1969.
3. Schmidt, P., Schoessler, J.P., Hill, R.M., Effects of hard contact lenses on the chloride ion of the tears. Amer. J. Optom., 51:84, 1974.
4. Hill, R.M., Osmotic edema associated with contact lens adaptation. J. Amer. Optom. Assoc., 46:897, 1975.
5. Terry, J.E., Hill., R.M., The osmotic variable. J. Amer. Optom. Assoc., 48:311, 1977.
6. Carney, L.G., Hill, R.M., Tear pH and the hard (PMMA) contact lens patient. Intern. Contact Lens Clinic, 3(1):27, 1976.
7. Moses, R.A., Adler's Physiology of the Eye, ed. 5. St. Louis: C.V. Mosby Co., 1970, p. 21.
8. Hill, R.M., Fatt, I., Oxygen measurements under a contact lens. Amer. Acad. Optom., 41:382, 1964.

Chapter Twenty-Four

PMMA and Its Environmental Variations

Could one-third cubic millimeter of water be of any substantial consequence in modern contact lens practice? If it happens to be that volume contained in the average PMMA contact lens, it could very well be, for that tiny amount, and most particularly its variations, may be the source of some of the most subtle disturbances these lenses can undergo. Clinically they show themselves as slight drifts in base curve, just-measureable changes in lens diameter, or, through stress adjustments, as optical aberrations.

Tracking Transitions

When such alterations do occur in practice, they generally progress so gradually that only patient signs and symptoms, or a very careful long-term reinspection, are likely to reveal them. In the research laboratory, however, monitoring techniques have become sufficiently refined that such changes can sometimes be detected within the very first soaking or wearing hours of a lens' service life.[1]

Using such methods, we can get a controlled view, for example, of what can happen to PMMA which is still "dry," but has become adjusted over a day or so to room (or office) level humidity, only to be placed abruptly into a saturated environment. Even when in a soaking chamber, as described in Figure 1, PMMA samples could be seen to absorb water

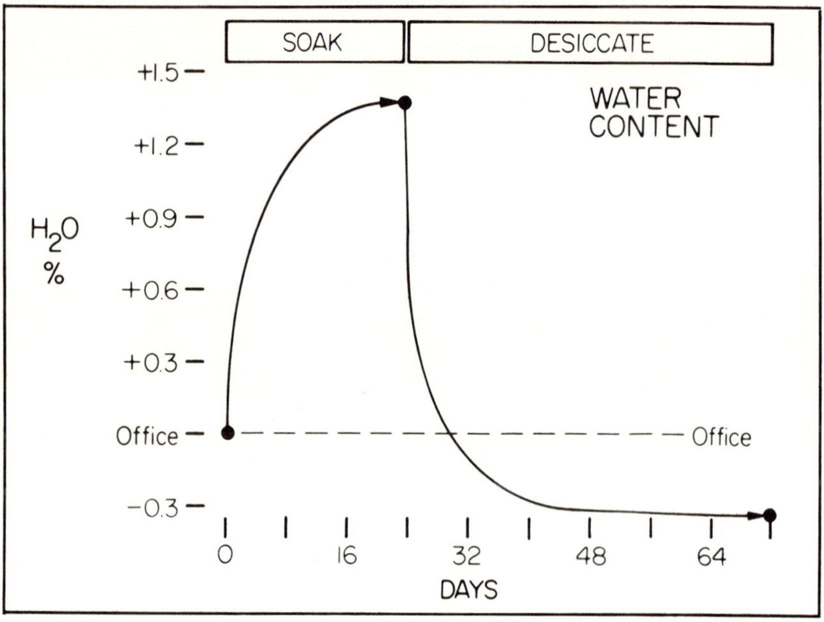

FIGURE 1. The average hydration changes of a group of 10 PMMA samples that were first soaked and then dried.

very rapidly at first but then finally to level off in 10 to 12 days, averaging a new weight gain of some 1.4 percent.

However, this water gain can be just as readily lost when PMMA is allowed to dry once again in the room atmosphere. If, as in Figure 1, this material is placed in a desiccation (drying agent) chamber, even more water can be forced from it.

Clinical Consequences

But it is the dimensional changes of PMMA secondary to these water variations that are the most clinically interesting. Some, like center thickness, appear to be almost completely reversible, while others, such as surface dimensions, may not. The resulting "hysteresis" (i.e., imperfect return, due for example to the release of casting or manufacturing stress) may eventually be great enough to become optically evident as irregular aberrations within the material.

While nearly all bodies register some change in response to their environments (e.g., the Eiffel Tower varies as much as six inches in height with the fluctuations of air temperature surrounding it), these changes are generally of little or no functional consequence. In contrast, a drift of just microns (millionths of a meter) between two bench marks scored on the

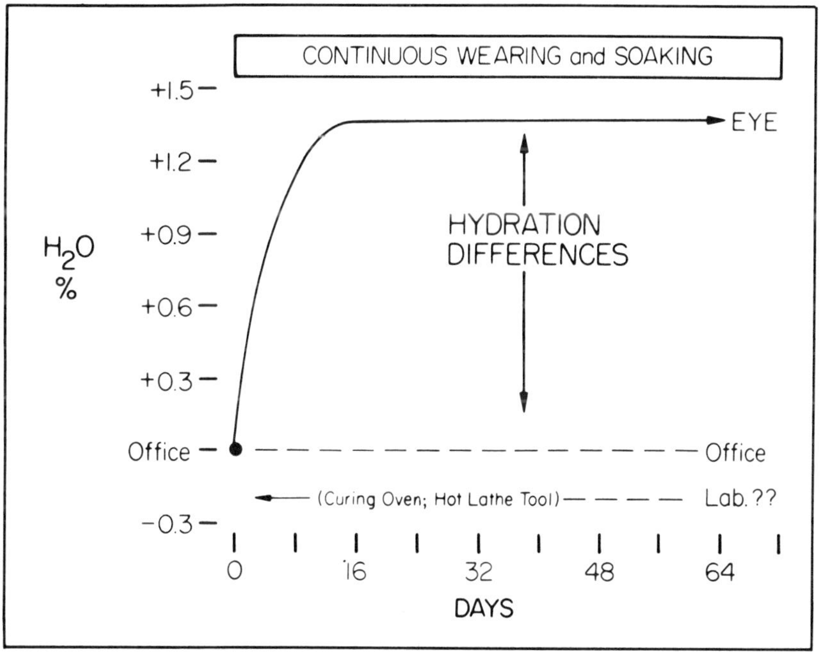

FIGURE 2. The several hydration levels a lens may assume in its lifetime, from the lowest (in the form of stock leaving the curing oven) to its functional highest (on the eye). The stable plateau shown assumes a regular soaking regimen whenever the lens is not being worn.

front surface of PMMA sample may correspond to optically significant disturbances progressing through its interior.

Particularly, then if a PMMA lens is routinely stored dry each night, it may be oscillating between two significantly different hydration levels. If kept soaked when not in the eye, however, it should reach a virtually stable state of hydration by about two weeks of service life and essentially remain there, as indicated in Figure 2. This would seem to be the optimum time to establish the most reliable verification measurements of such a lens on a routine recheck visit.

It should be noted that the hydration changes described above are, if anything, on the modest side, since (1) relatively thick PMMA samples were studied here, and of course the thinner a lens, the faster such changes will take place; and (2) the saturated water levels of certain PMMA types commonly used in contact lens practice today are now known to be as much as double those demonstrated here.[2]

References

1. Flower, F.C., and R.M. Hill, Polymethyl-methacrylate: Measures of hydration. *Amer. J. Optom.*, 49:935-937, 1972.
2. *Physiochemical Properties of Conventional Hard Plastic Contact Lenses.* New York: American National Standards Institute, Doc. Z80.6, 1976.

Chapter Twenty-Five

Oxygen Permeable Contact Lenses: How Convinced Is the Cornea?

Possibly the greatest physiological boon of this new material's era has been an increasing freedom the fitter has gained in the design and management of tear-oxygen "pumps." This has been the direct result of a "second source" of oxygen to the corneal surface: *gas transmission through the lens itself.* Although silicone rubber and certain of the hydrophilic materials have lead the way, several types of hard materials are now featuring this property as well.

But how "convinced" is the cornea?

One Way to Approach the Question

Figure 1 summarizes one method of observing the cornea's response to such materials. If, as shown in the upper part of the illustration, a cornea is exposed to air, it will reveal its "normal thirst" for oxygen by the rate it drains a small gas reservoir placed against its surface (note the "leisurely" slope on the small accompanying graph).

A contact lens, however, represents a barrier to oxygen approaching the eye, so immediately after wearing such a "test lens" (see the middle part of Figure 1), the cornea displays an increased "thirst" for oxygen (indicated now by the much more rapid exhaustion of the gas reservoir when placed against the cornea).

To carry this exercise just one step further, a goggle can be placed

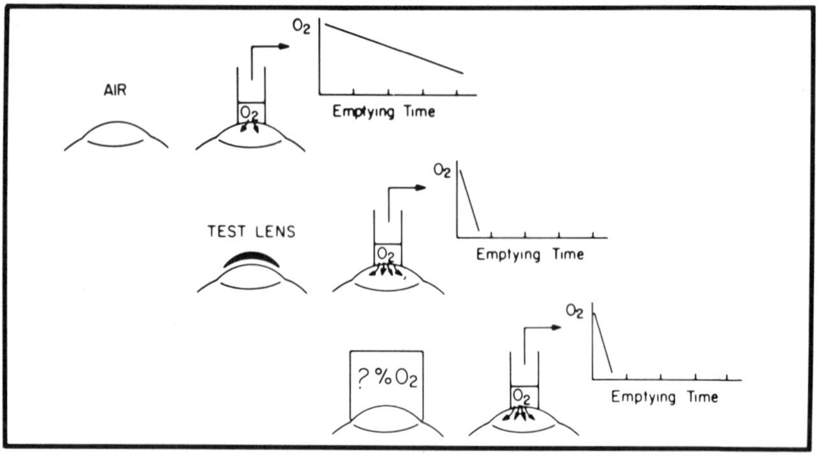

FIGURE 1. A means of observing the living cornea's response to an oxygen permeable contact lens.

over the eye and filled with different percentages of oxygen until that percentage producing the same corneal "thirst" as the "test lens" is found. We can then say that the "test lens" is found. We can then say that the "test lens" caused the cornea to behave as if it had been living in that percentage of oxygen. We call that percentage the *equivalent oxygen* performance of the lens.

A Quick Look at the Candidates

When one uses this method to "consult" the cornea, how do the various classes of contact lenses materials compare in their oxygen permeabilities?

The graphical format shown in Figure 2 allows us to answer the question in relation to that very important design factor: *lens thickness.* The utopian hope would of course be to find an ideal test lens which would cause the eye to respond as if there were no lens present, i.e. at the 21 percent level of oxygen on the graph.

But no existing lens has quite reached that mark; instead, the fitter has learned to strive for some skillfully crafted blend of mechanical pump and lens permeability. The several criteria drawn across this format are indications of the degree of "relief" the patient might gain from his dependence on a mechanical tear pump, should the permeability of the contact lens reach such levels.

Into Perspective

Figure 3 summarizes the equivalent oxygen performances of several hard

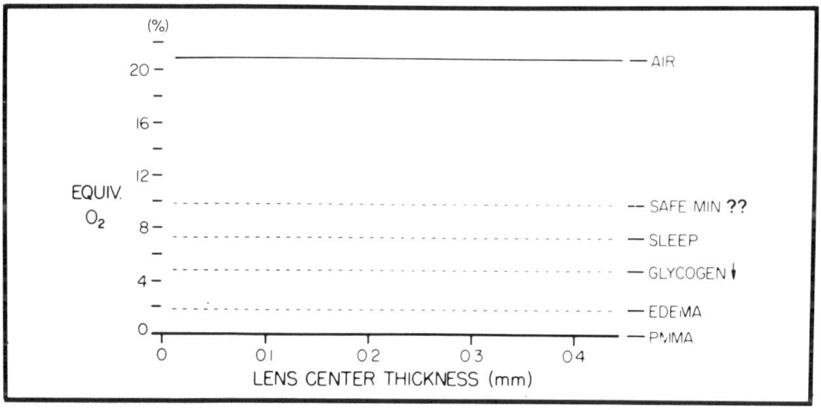

FIGURE 2. A format for comparing the equivalent *oxygen performances of various oxygen permeable contact lenses over a range of center thicknesses.*
—SAFE MINIMUM?: *Since even those levels present during sleep can result in minor corneal swelling, measurable on awakening, an arbitrary level a bit above, say at ten percent, might be taken for now as an exploratory estimate of the ideal minimum.*
—SLEEP (i.e., the prolonged lid closure condition): *Allows about seven to eight percent oxygen to reach the cornea.*[1]
—GLYCOGEN (sugar storage levels): *Oxygen levels in the epithelium begin to dissipate if there is less than five percent oxygen available.*[2]
—EDEMA: *Manifests as a measurable increase in corneal thickness if available oxygen falls below the level of 1.5 to 2.5 percent.*[3]
—PMMA: *Does not transmit a clinically significant amount of oxygen at any of these lens thicknesses.*[4]

and soft contact lens materials when examined at various center thicknesses.

While appraising such performances, however, at least two concepts should be kept in mind:

(1) Since any performance above the zero percent level will exceed the permeability of conventional PMMA (say 0.1mm or thicker), even those materials in the lower portion of the graph can contribute significantly to the success of a lens design—and may indeed be the materials of choice where they can offer other desired non-oxygen advantages as well.

(2) Those materials in the higher portion of the graph may be in a position to safely "sacrifice" a bit of oxygen performance through progressive improvements in their chemical make-up so that they might gain certain other clinically useful properties.

Just how such "bargains" will be struck between oxygen perfor-

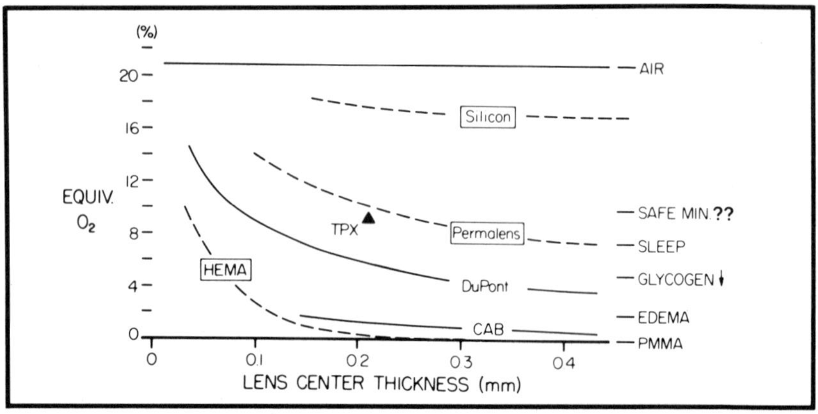

FIGURE 3. A comparison of the equivalent oxygen performance of several general classes of hard and soft contact lens materials. Performances will vary within a given class depending on differences in particular formulation and management techniques used by each manufacturing laboratory.

mance vs. other desirable prescription properties should prove, in the immediate future, to be one of the most fascinating aspects of this developing frontier.

References

1. Fatt, I., Freeman, R.D., and D. Lind, Oxygen tension distributions in the cornea: A re-examination. *Exp. Eye Res.*, 18:357-365, 1974.
2. Uniacke, C.A., Hill, R.M., Greenberg, M., and S. Seward, Physiological test for new contact lens materials. *Amer. J. Optom.*, 49:329-332, 1972.
3. Polse, K., and R.B. Mandell, Critical oxygen tension at the corneal surface, *Arch. Ophthal.*, 84(4):505-508, 1970.
4. *Physicochemical Properties of Conventional Hard Plastic Contact Lenses*, Z80.6-1976. New York: American Standards Institute, p. 7.

Chapter Twenty-Six

A Rare "Taste" for HEMA

Among those many surprises that the introduction of HEMA was to bring to the contact lens practitioner was the concept that this material in ordinary saline could support organism growth.

One of the most effective at this lens-destroying art was a fungus group called *Aspergillus*. But how common is this organism? How fast does it grow? What does it look like? Does it have pathological potential, and if so, what is our clinical protection?

An Invitation to "Dinner"

To explore those questions, a variety of the fungus* was invited directly onto an otherwise sterile HEMA surface, and that lens with its culture was then sealed in an observation container and allowed to remain for several days at room temperature.[1]

Figure 1 is a view of the lens surface after seven days of those conditions. The colony is seen to be well established at this site with hyphae ("tentacles") extending in all directions. A closer view of those

*This culture was *Aspergillus fumagatus* (ATCC 16424), which had been grown on Sabaroud agar slants. Sterile HEMA lenses of 38.6 percent water content (Bausch & Lomb) were used to receive the saline-suspended spores of this organism. The inoculated lenses were then sealed in a petri dish containing nonnutrition ion agar No. 2 and were maintained at room temperature.[1]

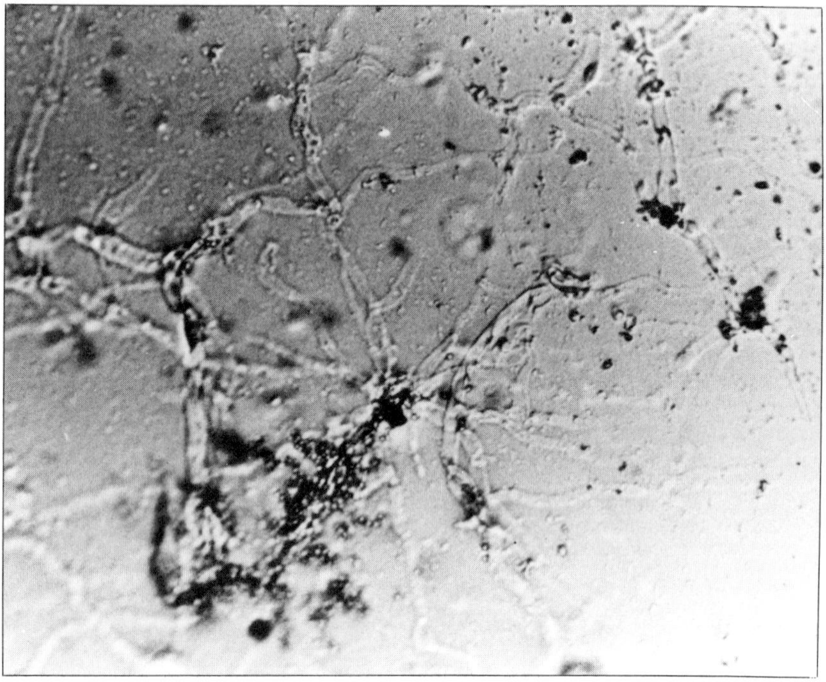

FIGURE 1. Fungal colony on the surface of a HEMA lens following seven days of growth at room temperature.

hyphae is shown in Figure 2.

Cross sections of the lens examined later revealed that growth had extended down into the lens interior as well. The "glove fit" of the HEMA around the penetrating hyphae suggested that the organism was enzymatically "eating" its way through the lens material.

Clinical Considerations

Although this organism is a fairly common one in the environment, the eye normally has quite adequate protection against it. It is under the unusual conditions, however, of corneal trauma (e.g., epithelial damage due to a particle caught under the lens) that such infection finds its chance, particularly if the lens is supporting an active colony readily at hand. Keratitis, conjunctivitis, and even orbital infections due to *Aspergillus* have all been recorded in the literature.

The development of any curious spot on a lens, then, should not go unheeded. While under the normally prescribed heat care procedures for HEMA lenses such organisms, including *Candida albicans* (another fun-

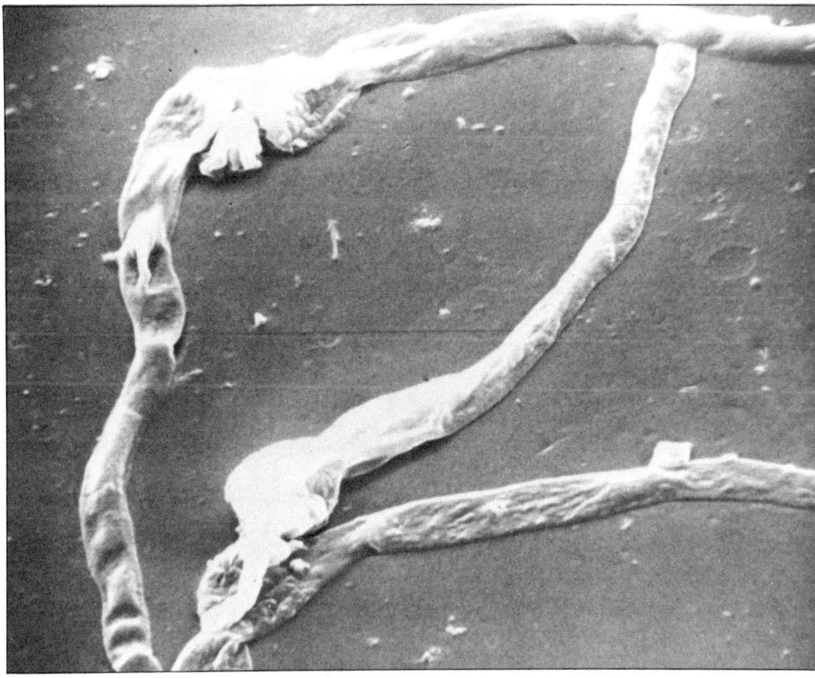

FIGURE 2. An enlarged view of fungal hyphae ("tentacles") on a HEMA lens surface.

gus), appear to be effectively killed,[2] the possibility of reinfection of the lens must be considered also.

Patient Management

These hygienic measures, however, are only effective, of course, when the patient carries them out. Herein, then, lie two basic responsibilities of the practitioner: (1) to train each patient carefully in the daily inspection and regular care of their lenses (heat or chemical, as appropriate) and (2) to emphasize the importance for bringing the lens in for inspection (and if need be, replacement) should surface changes appear. Only then can the health and best visual interests of the patient be assured.

References

1. Filippi, J.A., Pfister, R.M., Hill, R.M., Penetration of hydrophilic contact lenses by *Aspergillus fumagatus. Amer. J. Optom.*, 50:553-557, 1973.

2. Mote, E.M., Fillippi, J.A., Hill, R.M., Does heating arrest organisms in hydrophilic cases? *J. Amer. Optom. Assoc.*, 43:302-304, 1972.

Chapter Twenty-Seven

To Pasteurize, Sanitize, Asepticize, Sterilize . . .Or Just Disinfect?

As illustrated by the title, the *jargon jungle* of hydrophilic lens care represents one of the most confusing, even ominous, aspects of contact lens practice faced by the fitter today. For when delivering a prescription system to his patient which is described by one of those terms, what, in fact, is he promising? Table 1 offers the reader some clinical guidelines toward that answer.[1,2,3,4]

Probing the Inner Sanctums

But how close do various heat care systems come to satisfying such definitions?

The earliest approved hydrophilic care system was based on the Bausch & Lomb Aseptor® unit. Figure 1 gives a "lens-eye view" of that process, i.e., from inside the case, as recorded from a tiny electronic thermometer contained there. As can be seen, about 10 to 12 minutes were required for the maximum temperature, 96 degrees centigrade (or just under boiling) to be reached. After being maintained at that temperature for about 20 minutes, the contents of the case then began the cooling phase of the cycle.[5] In an operational sense, such a heating profile could be taken as a clinical definition of what has been called "asepticization," but, by definition of intent, this process appears to fit the more classical meaning of "disinfection" as well.

TABLE 1
Abstracted Definitions of Contact Lens Care Terms.[14]

Term	Definition
Asepticize	A "procedure of obtaining a pathogen-free solution"
Disinfect	To "free of pathogenic organisms or to render them inert"
Pasteurize	To "kill most species of pathogenic bacteria . . ."
Sanitize	To "clean and sterilize . . ."
Sterilize	"Any process, physical or chemical that destroys all forms of life"

Recently, the more absolute ("to destroy all forms of life") concept of sterilizing has been proposed as part of the home-care regime. To achieve this effect (i.e., for a substance such as rubber, and thus presumably for a hydrophilic contact lens), a temperature of 121 degrees centigrade should be maintained for a minimum of 15 minutes with an associated pressure of 15 pounds per inch.[2]

The average performance curve for one such instrument,* investigated by the same methods as above, is shown in Figure 2. Certainly, the temperature requirements of the definition are being very adequately met, and although the pressure within the case was not directly measured here, such temperatures could not be reached without substantial positive pressure within the case. Consistency of performance is critically important here; i.e., of the 10 cycles monitored for this system, did the coolest of them maintain 121 degrees centigrade for 15 minutes? As Figure 3 indicates, it just did.[6]

Causes for Compromise

If home sterilizing is, then, a reality, why settle for anything less? Two practical factors to consider in that answer are: (1) that certain materials have sufficiently low softening temperatures that repeated exposures to sterilization conditions may affect the prescription properties of such lenses; and (2) that repeated exposure of certain lenses containing polyvinylpyrrolidone (PVP) to those conditions may cause a progressive loss of that substance from them. One result of such a chemical alteration may be a significant reduction of water-holding capability.

*Durasoft Autoclave Sterilizer, model 205-50.

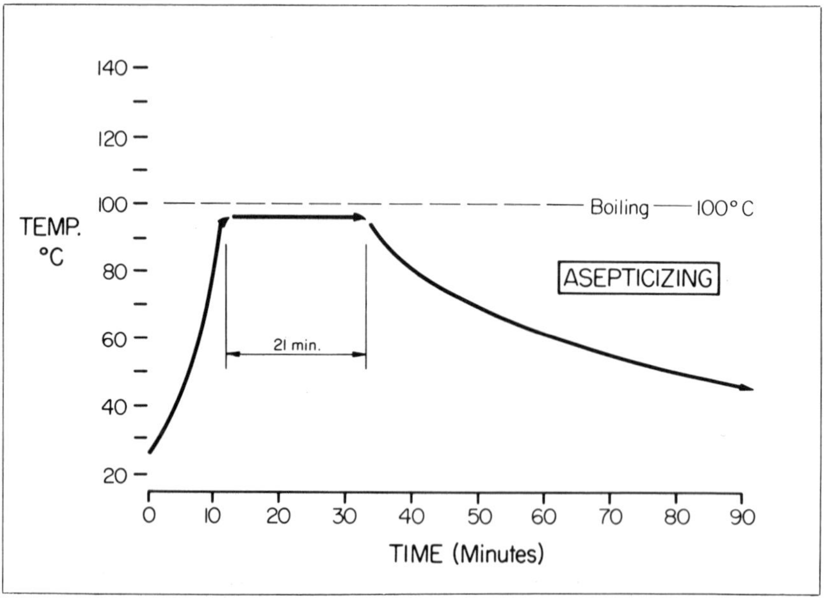

FIGURE 1. The average heating cycle temperatures measured for an "asepticizing" contact lens care unit.

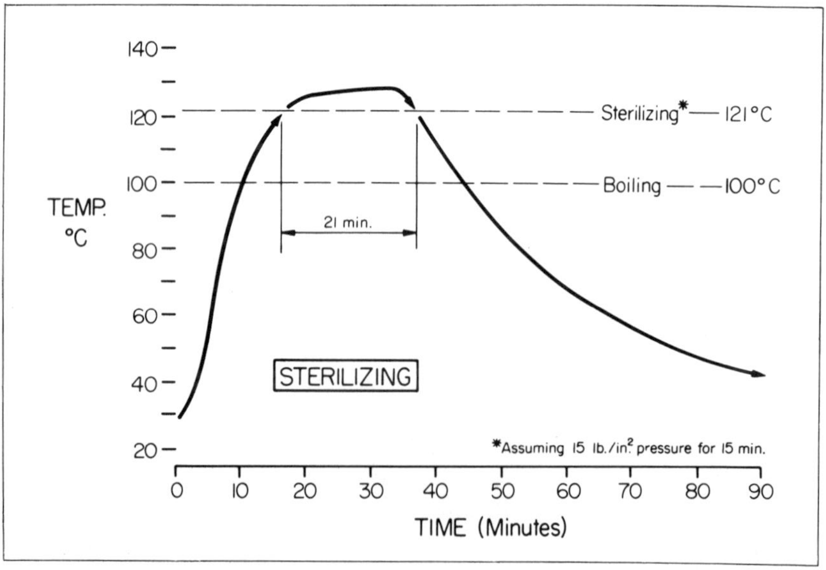

FIGURE 2. The average heating cycle temperatures measured for a "sterilizing" contact lens care unit. (High and lows shown in Figure 3.)

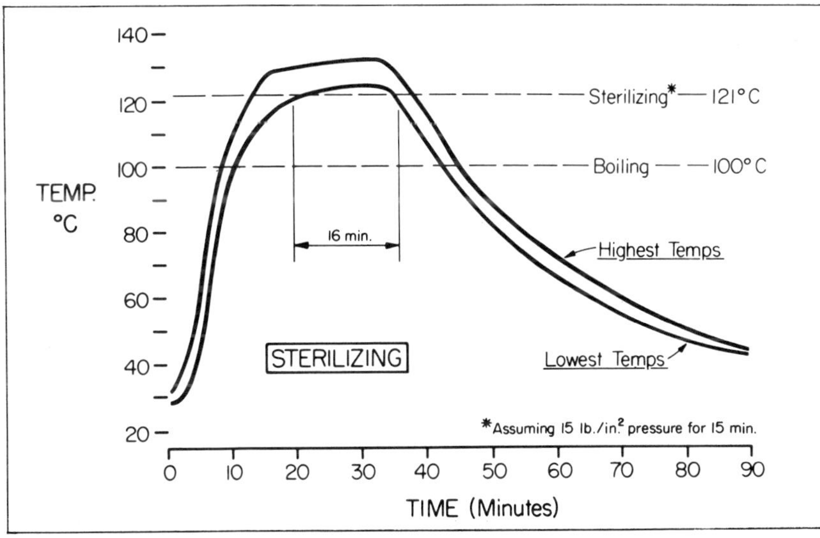

FIGURE 3. The high and low temperature range measurements for the "sterilizing" unit which is described in Figure 2.

Other Alternatives

Although both of the heating processes described here have so far proved clinically adequate from the microbiological point of view (and indeed, even "dry-heat" variations are now being explored) a spirited search for improvements and alternatives continues. Amongst those most-desired objectives sought are: a shorter time cycle requirement, fewer mechanical steps, less potential for patient error, reduced physical and chemical damage to the lens and better "economics." Since all such goals are directed toward more consistent and efficacious lens care by the patient, their early realization remains high on the list of clinical priorities today.

References

1. *Symposium on Flexible Lenses,* J. Bitonte and R. Keates (eds.). St. Louis: C.V. Mosby Co., 1972, p. 30.
2. *Stedman's Medical Dictionary,* 2st ed. Baltimore, Md.: The Williams and Wilkins Co., 1966, p. 152.
3. *Dorland's Illustrated Medical Dictionary,* 25th ed. Philadelphia: W.B. Saunders Co., 1974, pp. 464, 1147, 1377.
4. Locather-Khorazo, D. and Seegal, B., *Microbiology of the Eye.* St. Louis: C.V. Mosby Co., 1972, p. 91.
5. Mote, E.M., Filippi, J.A. and R.M. Hill, Does heating arrest organisms in hydrophilic cases? *J. Amer. Optom. Assn.,* 43:302, 1972.
6. Snyder, A.C., Hill, R.M. and N.J. Bailey, Hydrophilics: Is home sterilizing a reality? *Contact Lens Forum* (to be published).

Chapter Twenty-Eight

How "Pure" are the Waters?

Surely in this new era of ophthalmically packaged "salines", the problems of "impure" water should be well past!

Yet, those who use salt and/or enzyme tablets still run the risk of purchased water damage to their hydrophilic contact lenses. So, how pure are the commercially obtainable "distilled" waters which they might use?

The Market Place

To explore that question, seven brands of distilled water (these words had to appear on the container label) were purchased from supermarket and drugstore outlets within a five day period. Their purities were measured by a precision conductivity meter (i.e. the more impurities present, the higher was the conductivity of a water sample.)

All of the waters tested, A through G, were compared with a *standard* water, which was triple distilled in glass and demineralized. Its total impurity rating was less than 0.1 parts per million (ppm) as indicated in Figure 1.

Often the word *purified* will appear as well on the container label, as in the case of water A in Figure 2. But as noted, water A contained some 11 times more impurities than our standard.

Waters B and C, in Figure 3, featured two further characteristics which *may* appear on such labels: the "famous tradename" and the

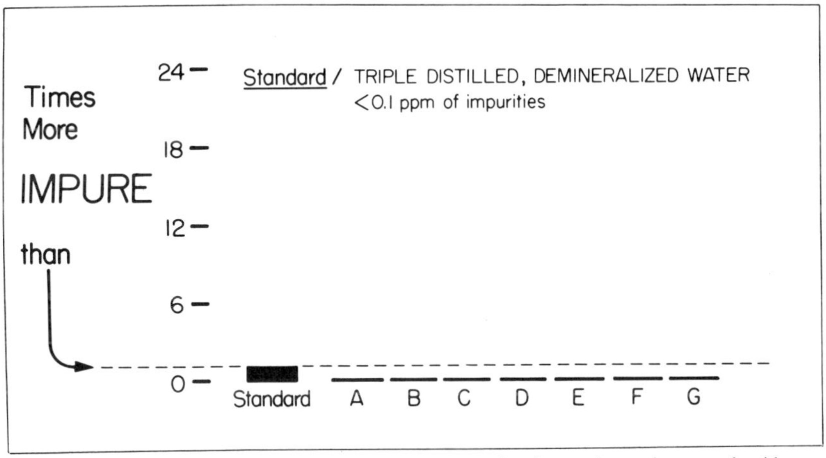

FIGURE 1. Quality level of the water standard used in this study (1 on the relative scale at the left = 0.2 micro-ohms/cm).

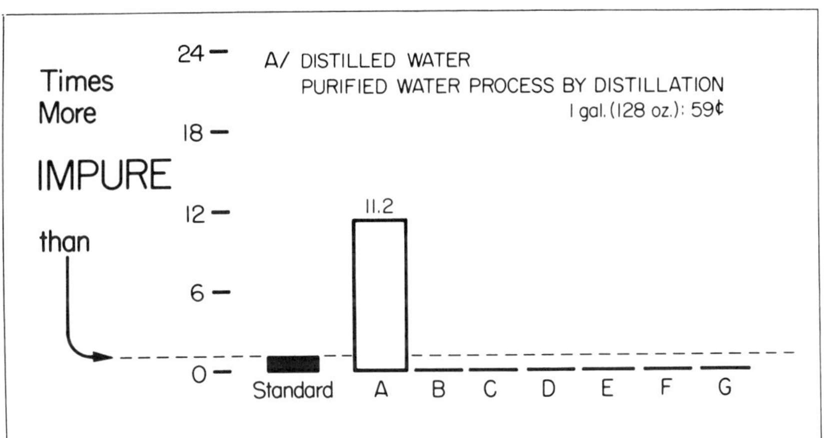

FIGURE 2. The relative performance of a water described as "purified", (A).

"state permit number." While the precise impact of those factors on product quality remains uncertain, at least here, the findings for these two waters were gratifyingly closer to our standard.

In fact, one could almost believe, with regard to state permit numbers, that this is one of those rare cases where "more is better," as suggested by the even superior quality of water D in Figure 1. But alas, just one state permit number of the "right" kind may be equally good, as noted for water E in that Figure, (especially when accompanied by the words "purified water, U.S.P."[1]).

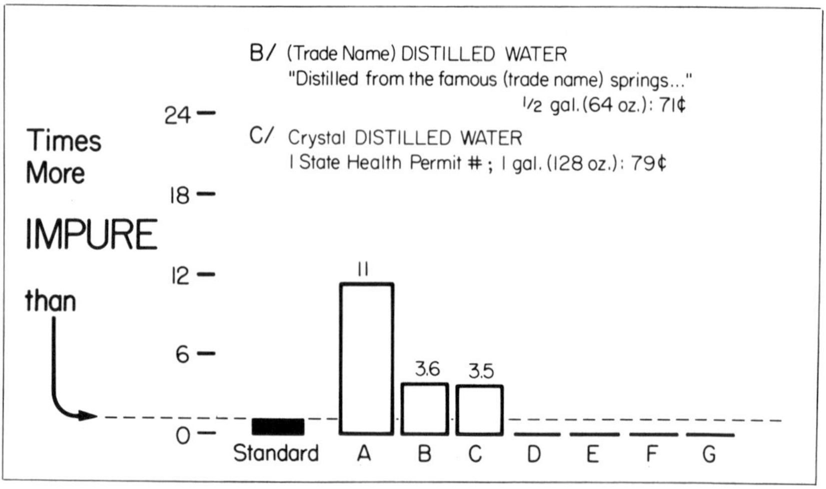

FIGURE 3. An example of a water with a "famous" trade-name and origin (B), as well as one with a state permit number (C).

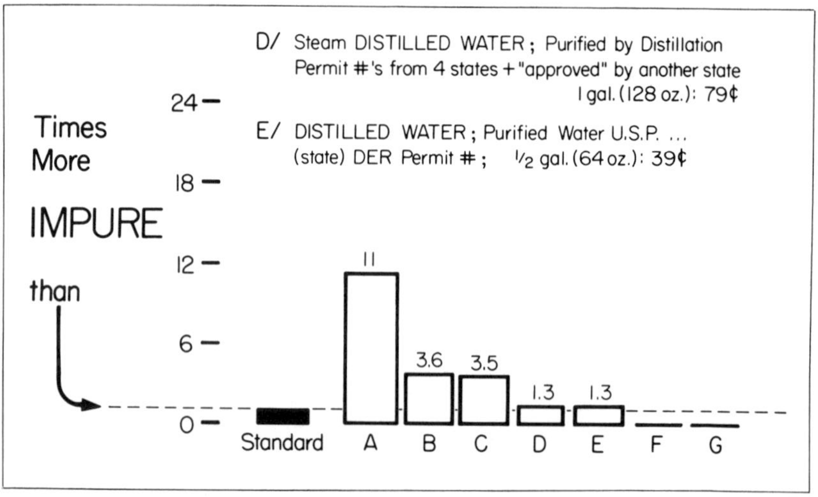

FIGURE 4. An example of a water with permit numbers from four different states, and an approval from another (D), as well as one with "purified water, U.S.P." on the label (E).

Most interesting to the practitioner however (and clearly astonishing as well), will be the two waters, F and G, shown in Figure 5. Apart from a low impurity claim, their most distinctive label feature was a direct recommendation for their use with *CONTACT LENSES.* But it appears, in these two cases at least, that neither that recommendation nor the

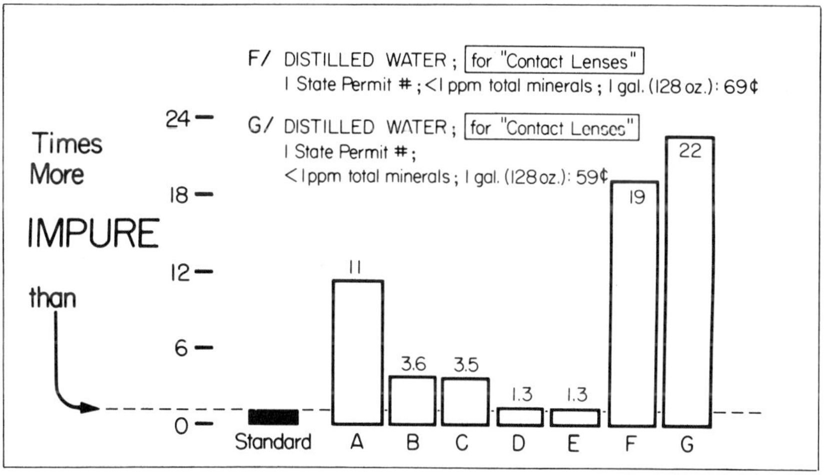

FIGURE 5. Two waters specifically recommended for CONTACT LENS use (F and G).

presence of a state permit number was of very positive assistance.

Are Ophthalmically Packaged Waters Better?

Although "red eye response" and "cost" have been two areas of practical concern associated with ophthalmically packaged waters, they do commonly offer U.S.P. guidelines and/or F.D.A. traceability should contamination or a formulation error occur. But of course such problems remain esoteric to the average patient—until they happen.

In the interim then, it is the practitioner's obligation to remain alert to problems which may stem from certain commercially purchased waters, and to guide each patient's lens care accordingly.

Reference

1. For U.S.P. definitions of water types (for example "purified"), see:
The Pharmacopeia of the U.S.A. (most recent revision) U.S.P. 7630 Montgomery Ave. Bethesda Md. 20014, Publ. and Distr.: Mack Printing Co. Easton PA 18042.

Chapter Twenty-Nine

Nine Lives of a Gel-Lens

One of the most fascinating and widely varying features among contact lens candidates is the "cleanness" of their tears. While the lower tear prism (i.e. those tears spanning from the lower lid margin across to the corneal and conjunctival surfaces) of some are crystal clear, others will contain an almost indescribable collection of protein coagulant, bubbles, cell clumps and other assorted forms of "rubbish."

But how *little* tear content is enough to trigger an enduring film on a lens surface?

Declining Fortunes

Beyond the obvious clinical variables of composition, concentration and tear turn-over time, there is, of course, the most unpredictable factor of all: *patient care of the lens*—in particular, its nature and its frequency.

Suppose, for reasons of haste, carelessness, or lack of fitter reinforcement, the patient omits just one step: *the gentle dislodging of tear debris from the lens surfaces.* If this brief procedure is not carried out regularly and with care, that most unique feature, *oxygen passage,* especially of the hydrophilic ultra-thin, is placed at risk.[1,2]

To demonstrate, suppose we monitor in Figure 1, the averaged histories of six HEMA (38.6% water content) ultra-thin lenses as they passed through the following sequence:

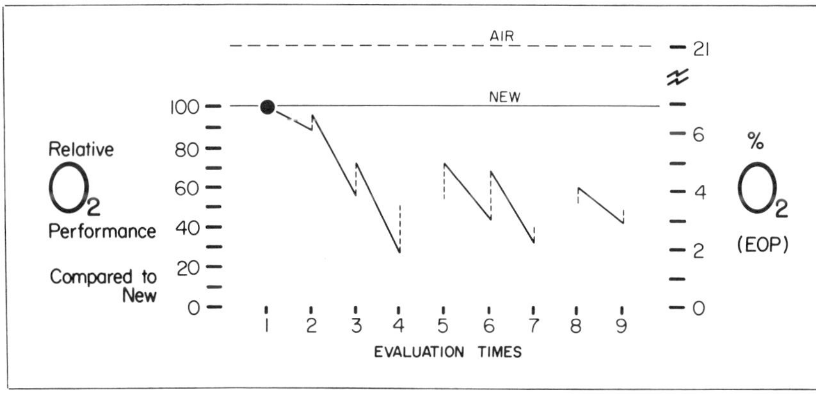

FIGURE 1. The effects of repeated protein coating and heat cycles on the oxygen performances of 6 ultra-thin lenses (averaged here), before mechanical cleaning (lower points) and after mechanical cleaning (upper points) at each evaluation time.

(1) First, their oxygen performances (equivalent oxygen percentages or EOP's) were measured when brand new. Their averaged value was nearly 7%, as compared to 21% oxygen contained in the air (see the first "evaluation time").

(2) Each lens was then dipped in a saline solution containing 1% human protein (active albumin) and without rinsing or cleaning, it was put through a heat cycle, peaking and holding at 96°C for 20 minutes.[3] This protein dip-heating procedure was repeated six times after which the oxygen performances of the lenses were measured again (see the lower point at the second "evaluation time").

(3) Each of the lenses was then mechanically cleaned in fresh saline, and its oxygen performance measured once more where some improvement can be noted (upper point at the second "evaluation time").

Steps (2) and (3) were repeated over and over again, until a total of 48 "protein dip-heating" procedures, interspersed with 8 mechanical cleanings, had been completed (i.e. through to "evaluation nine").

But notice as "evaluation nine" was approached, the restoration effect (i.e. the dashed line lengths representing the re-elevations of oxygen performance) tended to diminish, and even the post-cleaned performances remained well below the "new" condition level of these lenses.

Break-Away Points

There is however, one other phenomenon taking place along this sequence. In Figure 1 it is indicated by interruptions in the "sawtooth"

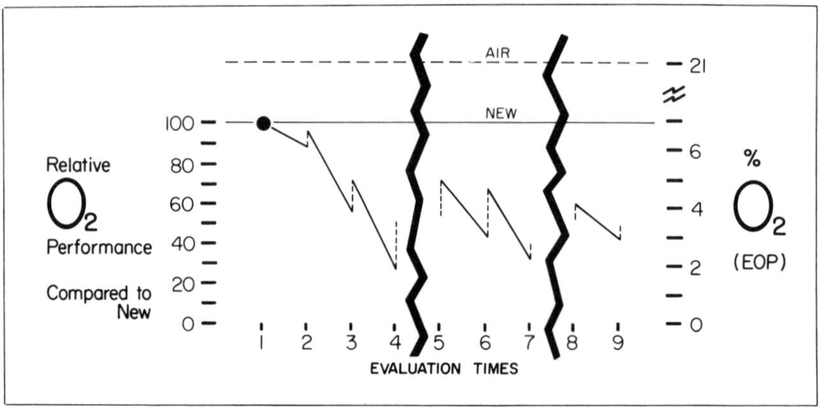

FIGURE 2. The same data as shown in Figure 1, but with the discontinuities in oxygen performance (coating "break-away" points from the lens surfaces) emphasized.

pattern (i.e. between evaluation times 4 and 5, and between 7 and 8 as well). From observations of the lenses, these discontinuities appear to be "break-away" points, at which times the protein coating seems to have become sufficiently rigid that it fractured from the lens surfaces during flexure. As emphasized stylistically in Figure 2, it is at such times that the oxygen performance (with fair synchrony throughout the group) improves significantly, giving, very likely in the clinical world, the patient an "unearned" reprieve. But even those "spontaneous" recoveries seem to become less and less restorative as this parade of neglect continues.

So, it would appear then, particularly in those cases with demonstrated histories of lens coating, that regular mechanical care should be taken as a *most fundamental step* toward preserving the "oxygen investment" in an ultra-thin. It is possibly, the very best argument a fitter can offer for the cause of continuous (daily) lens care.

References

1. Benjamin, W.J. and Hill, R.M. Ultra-Thins: The case for continuous care, *J. Amer. Optom. Assoc.* 51:277, 1980.
2. Benjamin, W.J. *Equivalent Oxygen Performance of Optical Polymers with Respect to Surface Coatings,* Thesis, M.S. degree, The Ohio State University, Columbus, Ohio, 1979.
3. Mote, E.M., Filippi, J.A. and Hill, R.M. Does heating arrest organisms in hydrophilic cases: *J. Amer. Optom. Assoc. 43:302, 1972.*

Chapter Thirty

Spoilation and its Related Implications

Of the many methods in use for scaling surface spoilation, one of the most clinically comprehensive is the "Rudko" system.[1] It has the advantage of accounting for the *heaviness*, the *type* and the *extent* of surface accumulations.[a]

But can such surface evaluations be "translated" into other useful indexes of lens performance?

Combinations and Consequences

To explore this possibility, the surface signs associated with progressive protein build-up on 6 ultra-thin HEMA lenses was monitored and scaled using a modified Rudko system,[1] and their corresponding oxygen performances (equivalent oxygen percentages or EOP's) were measured as well.[2,3] To accelerate the deposit build-up process, each lens was dipped into a 1% solution (in saline) of human protein (albumin) just previous to being put through a heat cycle (holding at 96°C for 15 to 20 minutes). This protein dip-heat cycle sequence was applied repeatedly. Although the 1% protein concentration used here was a little above the normal tear average (0.6 to 0.8%), it is well within the province of many tear problem patients.

As indicated in Figure 1, the collective oxygen performances of these lenses averaged, when new (Rudko I), about 7% (compared to 21%

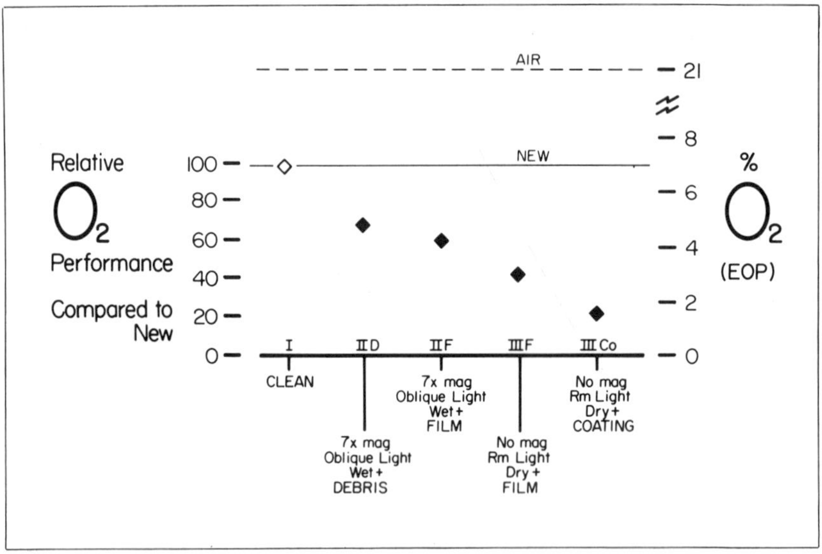

FIGURE 1. Relationships between lens surface appearance (see text), and oxygen performance, for a series of 6 HEMA ultra-thin lenses subjected to repeated cycles of human protein exposure and heat disinfection.

oxygen available directly from the air), an expected level for HEMA (38.6% water content) lenses of that average center thickness (0.06^{+}mm). But, as their degrees of spoilation advanced (even just using for convenience here the *heaviness* and *type* ratings of the Rudko system), their oxygen performance values can indeed, be seen to decline correspondingly.

A Critical Cut-off?

But how far along this spoilation scale is a lens likely to go before clinical performance begins to suffer?

By the time the IIF stage (see footnote a) has occurred, the relative

---

[a]Minimum observation conditions required for surface build-up evaluation*

HEAVINESS:	*I* = clean; *II* = oblique light, 7X magnification, wet surface; *III* = room light, no magnification, dry surface; *IV* = no magnification, wet or dry surface.
TYPE:	*C* = crystalline; *G* = granular; *F* = film; *P* = plaque; *D* = debris; *Co* = coating.
EXTENT:	*a* = 0 to 25%; *b* = 25 to 50%; *c* = 50 to 75% and *d* = 75 to 100% of the surface.

*Modified Rudko System (see Reference 1)

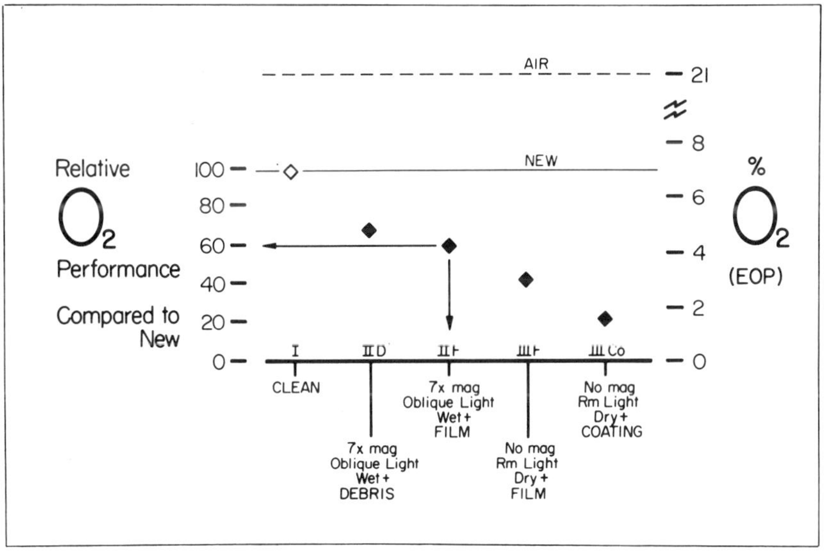

FIGURE 2. Same data as in Fig. 1, with a critical cut-off level for visual performance and comfort together with the associated surface appearance and oxygen performances of those lenses (arrows).

oxygen performance of such a lens will be reduced to about 60% of what it was when new, as shown in Figure 2. For ultra-thins, such as these, this would still correspond to about 4% oxygen (EOP), a level which should keep the cornea above the edema detection zone of Polse and Mandell (approximately 1.5 to 2.5%),[4] but would not allow it to maintain its full capacity of energy reserves.[5] A patient wearing such lenses would, in any event, very probably return to the fitter for reasons of reduced visual acuity or discomfort by that point.

In terms of dealing clinically then with the surface spiolation problem and its related implications, the most logical strategies would seem to be: (1) to frankly discourage contact lens candidates with excessively ladened and viscous tears, since functionally, the odds of success will run significantly against both fitter and patient over the long term; (2) to encourage regular, gentle mechanical cleaning by all wearers, but most especially by ultra thin patients who have an "oxygen investment" to protect; and (3) to realize the related implications of surface spoilation to other lens-eye factors, e.g. the energy reserves of the cornea, visual acuity, comfort, and very possibly even eye health.

References

1. Hathaway, R.A., *The Compatibility of a Hydrophilic Lens Polymer (HEMA) with the Human Tear Fluid,* M.S. Thesis, The Ohio State University, Columbus, Ohio 1976, pg. 48.
2. Benjamin, W.J., *Equivalent Oxygen Performance of Optical Polymers with Respect to Surface Coatings,* M.S. Thesis, The Ohio State University, Columbus, Ohio, 1979, pg. 14.
3. Benjamin, W.J. and Hill, R.M., Ultra-thins: The case for continuous care, *J. Amer. Optom. Assoc.,* 51:277, 1980).
4. Polse, K. and Mandell, R.B., Critical oxygen tension at the corneal surface, *Arch. Ophthal.* 84:505, 1970.
5. Uniacke, C.A., Hill, R.M., Greenberg, M. and Steward, S., Physiological tests for new contact lens materials, *Amer. J. Optom.* 49:329, 1972.